Renal Diet Coo

The Ultimate Healthy Guide to Stopping Kidney Disease and Avoiding Dialysis with Quick and Delicious Low Sodium and Potassium Recipes

Written By

Delilah Hooper

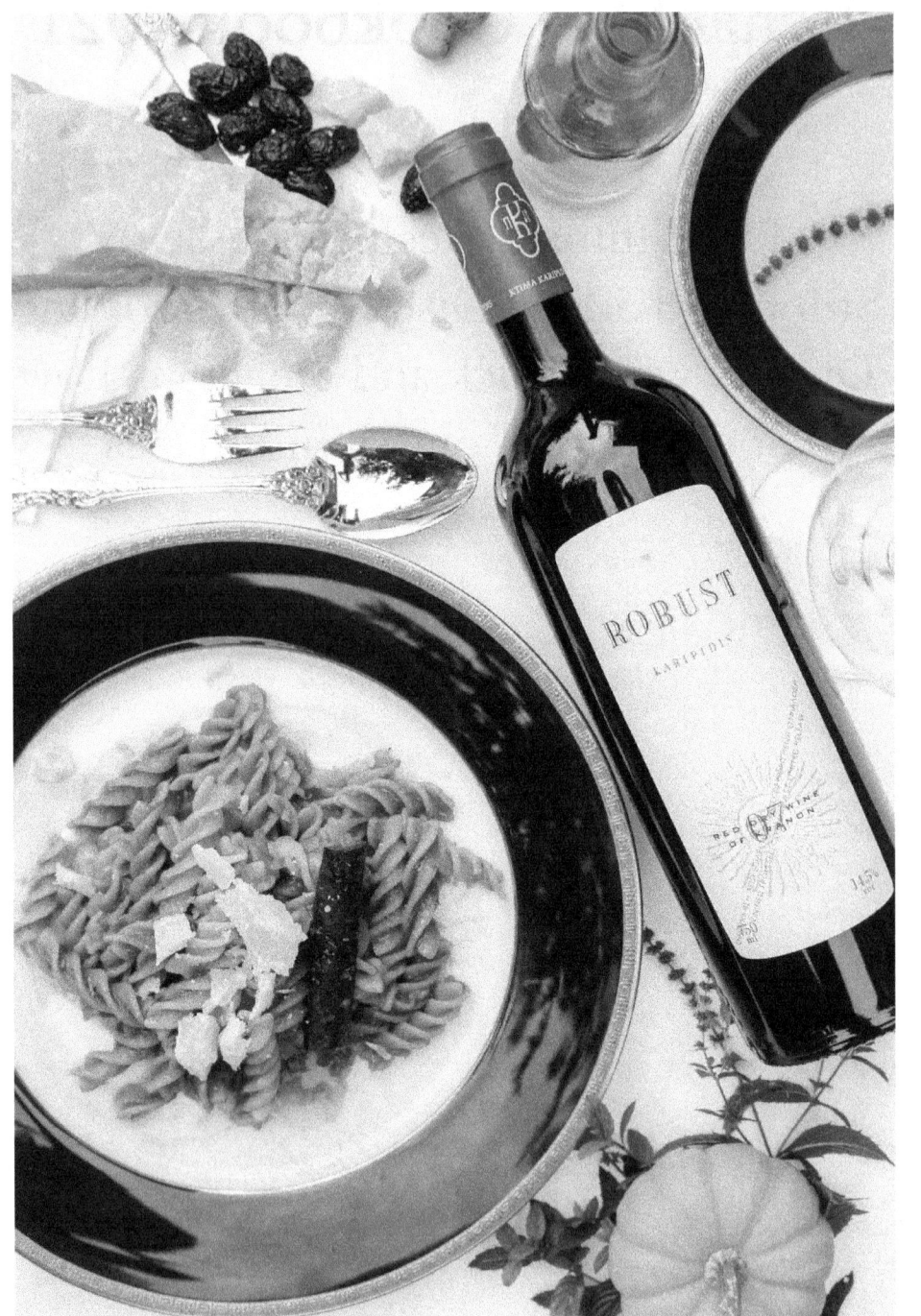

© Copyright 2021 - All rights reserved.

The content contained within this book may not be reproduced, duplicated or transmitted without direct written permission from the author or the publisher.

Under no circumstances will any blame or legal responsibility be held against the publisher, or author, for any damages, reparation, or monetary loss due to the information contained within this book. Either directly or indirectly.

Legal Notice:

This book is copyright protected. This book is only for personal use. You cannot amend, distribute, sell, use, quote or paraphrase any part, or the content within this book, without the consent of the author or publisher.

Disclaimer Notice:

Please note the information contained within this document is for educational and entertainment purposes only. All effort has been executed to present accurate, up to date, and reliable, complete information. No warranties of any kind are declared or implied. Readers acknowledge that the author is not engaging in the rendering of legal, financial, medical or professional advice. The content within this book has been derived from various sources. Please consult a licensed professional before attempting any techniques outlined in this book.

By reading this document, the reader agrees that under no circumstances is the author responsible for any losses, direct or indirect, which are incurred as a result of the use of information contained within this document, including, but not limited to, — errors, omissions, or inaccuracies.

Table of Contents

Introduction 9
Breakfast Recipes 13
    1. Tofu and Mushroom Scramble 14
    2. Italian Apple Fritters 16
    3. Turkey Breakfast Sausage 18
    4. Blueberry Smoothie Bowl 20
    5. Egg White and Pepper Omelets 22
    6. Chicken Egg Rolls 24
    7. Pork Bread Casserole 26
    8. Salmon Bagel Toast 28
Lunch Recipes 29
    9. Authentic Shrimp Wraps 30
    10. Loveable Tortillas 32
    11. Elegant Veggie Tortillas 34
    12. Delightful Pizza 36
    13. Winner Kabobs 38
    14. Tempting Burgers 40
    15. Caraway Cabbage And Rice 42
    16. Gratin Pasta With Watercress And Chicken 43
Dinner Recipes 45
    17. Ground Beef And Rice Soup 46
    18. Persian Chicken 48
    19. Eggplant and Red Pepper Soup 50
    20. Seafood Casserole 52
    21. Ground Beef and Rice Soup 54

22.	Couscous Burgers	56
23.	Baked Flounder	58
24.	Spicy Chicken	60

Snacks & Sides Recipes 63

25.	Eggplant Sandwich	64
26.	Date and Blueberry Muffins	66
27.	Cranberry and Lemon Cookies	68
28.	No Bake Oat Cookies	70
29.	Chocolate Coconut Quinoa Slices	72
30.	Pineapple Raspberry Parfaits	74

Desserts Recipes 75

31.	Simple Berry Sorbet	76
32.	Chocolate Mousse	77
33.	Keto Brownie	79
34.	Smooth Coffee Mousse	80
35.	Almond Bites	82
36.	Chocolate Cookies	83
37.	Chocolate Muffins	85

Smoothies & Drinks 87

38.	Dark Turnip Greens Smoothie	88
39.	Butter Pecan and Coconut Smoothie	89
40.	Fresh Cucumber, Kale and Raspberry Smoothie	90
41.	Fresh Lettuce and Cucumber-Lemon Smoothie	92
42.	Green Coconut Smoothie	93
43.	Instant Coffee Smoothie	94
44.	Keto Blood Sugar Adjuster Smoothie	96

Salads 97

45.	Chestnut Noodle Salad	98

46.	Cranberry Broccoli Salad	99
47.	Balsamic Beet Salad	101
48.	Shrimp Salad	102
49.	Chicken Pomegranate Salad	104
50.	Egg Celery Salad	106
Conclusion		**107**

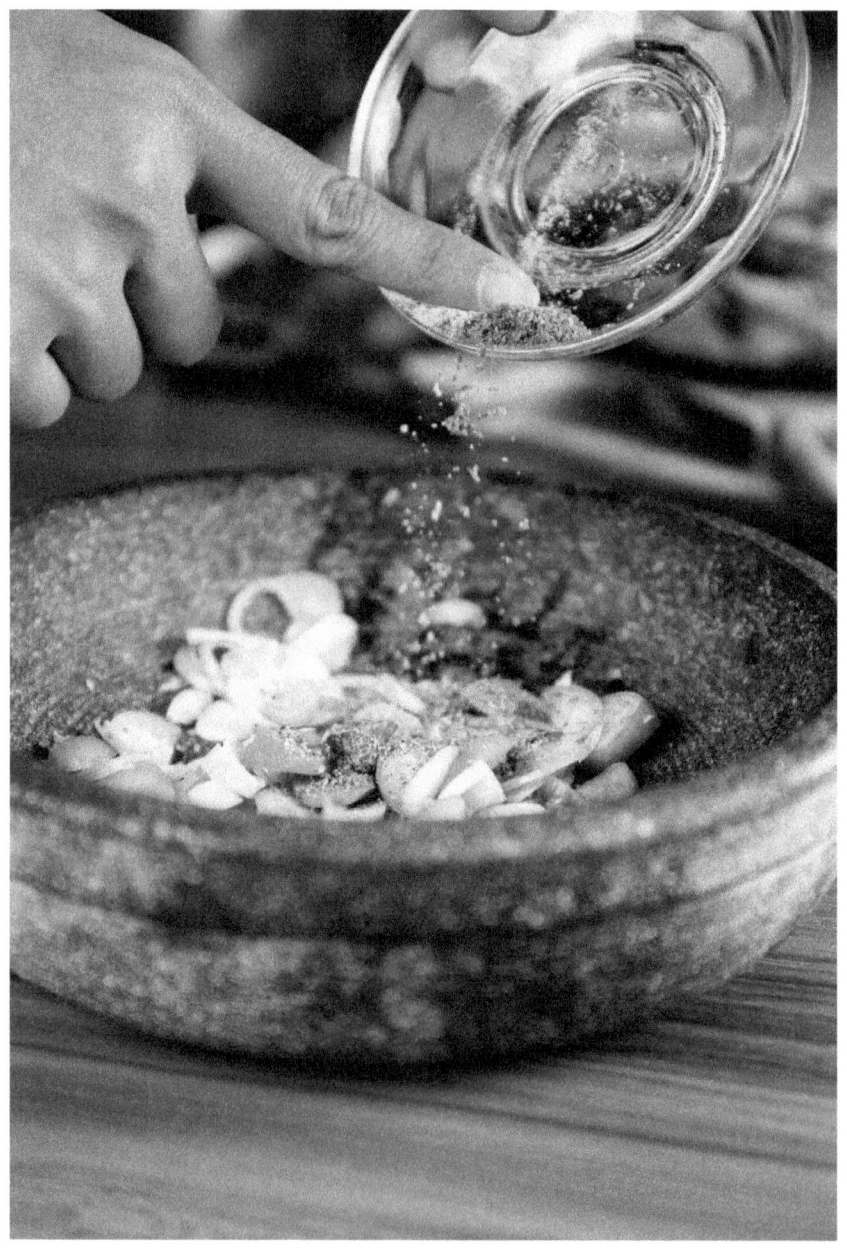

Introduction

Despite their tiny size, the kidneys perform a number of functions which are vital for the body to be able to function healthily.

These include:
- Filtering excess fluids and waste from the blood
- Creating the enzyme known as renin which regulates blood pressure
- Ensuring bone marrow creates red blood cells
- Controlling calcium and phosphorus levels through absorption and excretion

Unfortunately, when kidney disease reaches a chronic stage, these functions start to stop working. However, with the right treatment and lifestyle, it is possible to manage symptoms and continue living well. This is even more applicable in the earlier stages of the disease. Tactlessly, 10% of all adults over the age of 20 will experience some form of kidney disease in their lifetime. There are a variety of different treatments for kidney disease, which depend on the cause of the disease.

Possible causes are outlined below:

- DIABETES: In the United States and other countries where the 'Standard American Diet' runs rampant, the number one leading cause of kidney disease is high blood pressure and Type 2 diabetes. Both of these diseases are either completely preventable or at least treatable and once the root issue has been treated, kidney disease issues can also dissipate.

- GLOMERULONEPHRITIS: Damage to the glomeruli (the filters in your kidneys), impairs the kidneys' ability to filter waste materials. This can be caused by damage to the immune system and if this is the case, can be treated with medication. It is either experienced for a short period of time (acute glomerulonephritis), or for a longer period of time (chronic). In chronic cases, further problems can arise such as high blood pressure, organ damage and later chronic kidney disease.

- ACUTE RENAL FAILURE/ACUTE KIDNEY INJURY: Sudden damage or failure of the kidney can be caused by a rapid loss of blood to the kidneys, sepsis or even severe dehydration. Infection, poison and some medicines are also known to lead to acute kidney issues.

- SUDDEN BLOCKAGE: Kidney stones, tumors, injuries and an enlarged prostate in men can stop urine from passing through the kidneys as it should. This can cause swelling in the lower extremities, a loss of appetite, vomiting or nausea, extreme tiredness, restlessness, feelings of confusion, or even an acute pain beneath the ribs (known as flank pain).

- ECLAMPSIA: This can be experienced during pregnancy when the placenta doesn't function as it should do,
creating high blood pressure and sometimes leading to kidney problems.

- BREAKDOWN OF MUSCLE TISSUE: Under extreme pressure, for example when running a marathon or undergoing other feats of massive exertion, the body starts to break down muscle tissue after it has used all other available fuel. If this continues unchecked, too much of the protein known as myoglobin will ultimately end up in the bloodstream, putting undue strain on the kidneys and potentially leading to further implications.

- IMMUNE SYSTEM: Common immune system diseases that can lead to kidney issues include lupus, hepatitis C, hepatitis B, HIV, and aids. These can lead to what is known as chronic kidney disease (any form of kidney disease that lasts for three months or longer). Sometimes the sufferer of the immune disease will not experience the symptoms of the kidney disease until it reaches a chronic stage; this can be dangerous as it is a lot harder to manage once it has reached this level.

- EXTREME URINARY TRACT INFECTIONS: Urinary tract infections that occur within the kidneys rather than the bladder are known as pyelonephritis and occur when a traditional urinary tract infection remains untreated long enough for it to spread into the upper urinary tract system. This can cause scarring in the kidneys which can lead to severe flaws in kidney functioning.

- STREPTOCOCCAL INFECTIONS: Commonly known as a strep infection, this bacterium can infect the throat as well as various layers of the skin, the middle ear, the sinuses or even in a more severe case, a widespread vicious rash known as scarlet fever. This bacterium is known to result in the glomeruli (individual filters in the kidneys) becoming infected.

- POLYCYSTIC KIDNEY DISEASE: This type of kidney disease is typically passed down from parent to child and causes cysts filled with fluid to form on the kidneys themselves.

- BIRTH DEFECTS: Depending on the severity of the defect, kidney disease could form simply because the kidneys do not function correctly or because of an obstruction in the urinary tract before birth.

Breakfast Recipes

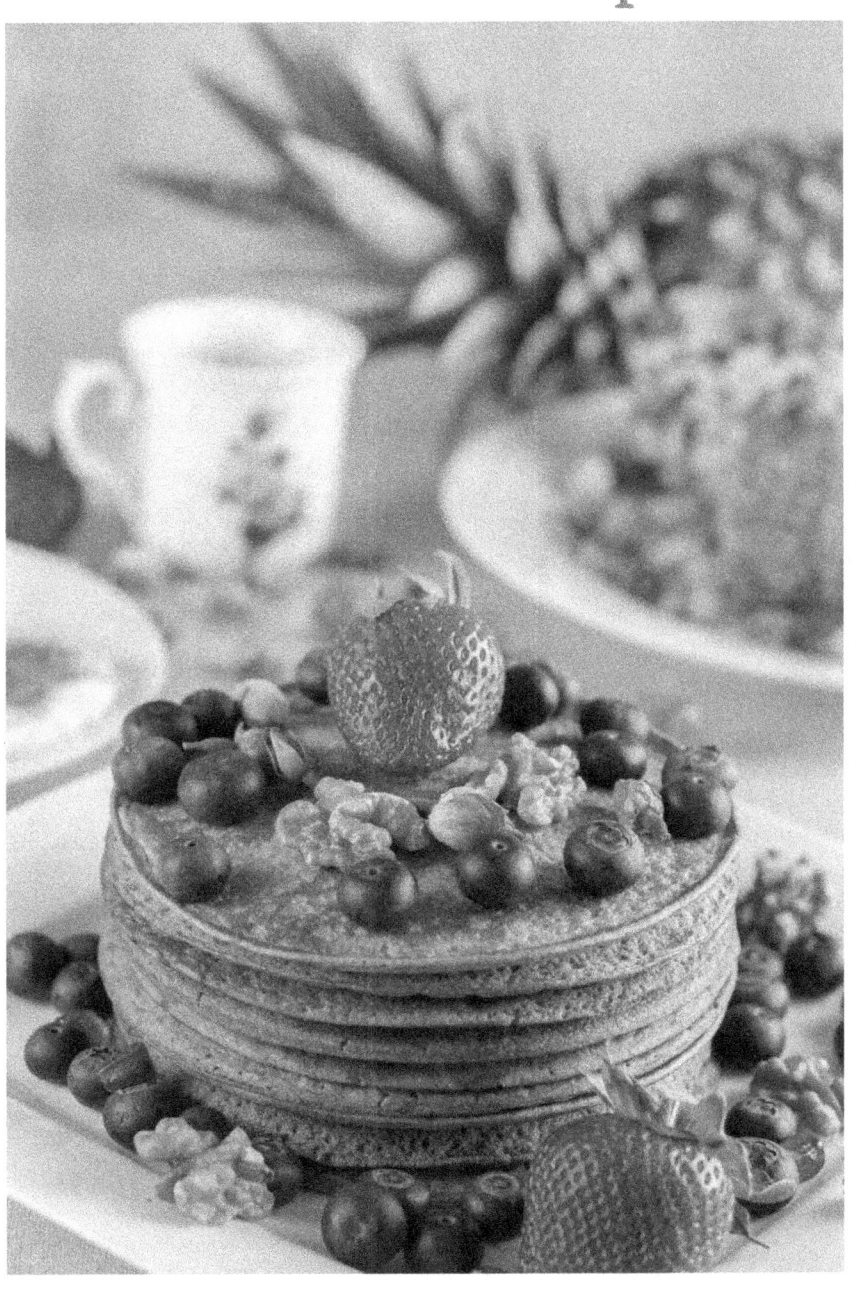

1. Tofu and Mushroom Scramble

Preparation Time: 5 minutes | *Cooking Time*: 8 minutes | *Servings*: 2

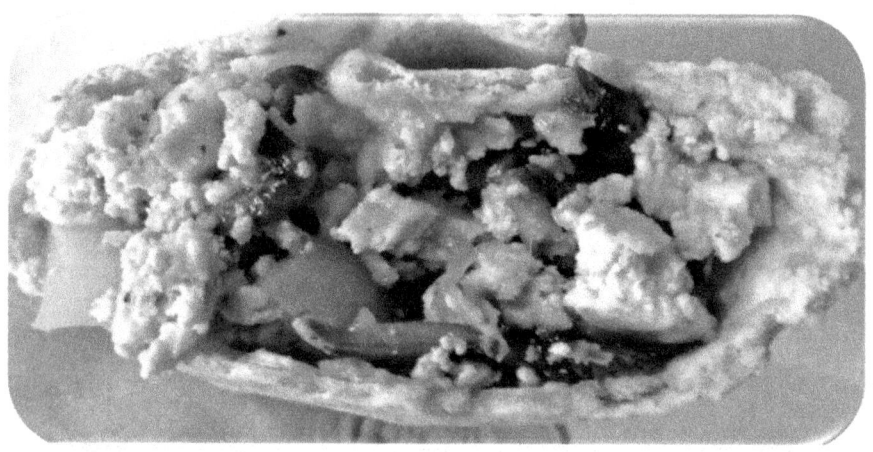

Ingredients:

- ½ cup of sliced white mushrooms
- ⅓ cup medium firm tofu, crumbled
- 1 tbsp of chopped shallots
- ⅓ tsp turmeric
- 1 tsp of cumin
- ⅓ tsp of smoked paprika
- ½ tsp of garlic salt
- Pepper
- 3 tbsp of vegetable oil

Directions:

Heat the oil in a medium frying pan and sauté the sliced mushrooms with the shallots until softened (around 3-4 minutes) over medium to high heat.

Add the tofu pieces and toss in the spices and the garlic salt.

Toss lightly until tofu and mushrooms are nicely combined. Serve warm.

Nutrition	Calories	Fat	Carbs	Protein	Sodium	Phosphorus	Potassium
	220	23g	2.5g	3g	223mg	68mg	135mg

2. Italian Apple Fritters

Preparation Time: 5 minutes | *Cooking Time:* 8 minutes | *Servings:* 4

Ingredients:

- 2 large apples, seeded, peeled and thickly sliced in circles
- 3 tbsp of corn flour
- ½ tsp of water
- 1 tsp of sugar
- 1 tsp of cinnamon
- Vegetable oil (for frying)
- Sprinkle of icing sugar or honey

Directions:

In a small bowl, combine the corn flour, water and sugar to make your batter.

Deep the apple rounds into the corn flour mix. Heat enough vegetable oil to cover half of the pan's surface over medium

to high heat. Add the apple rounds into the pan and cook until golden brown.

Transfer into a shallow dish with absorbing paper on top and sprinkle with a bit of cinnamon and icing sugar.

Nutrition	Calories	Fat	Carbs	Protein	Sodium	Phosphorus	Potassium
	183	6g	17g	0.5g	3mg	12mg	100mg

3. Turkey Breakfast Sausage

Preparation Time: 3 minutes | Cooking Time: 6 minutes | Servings: 6

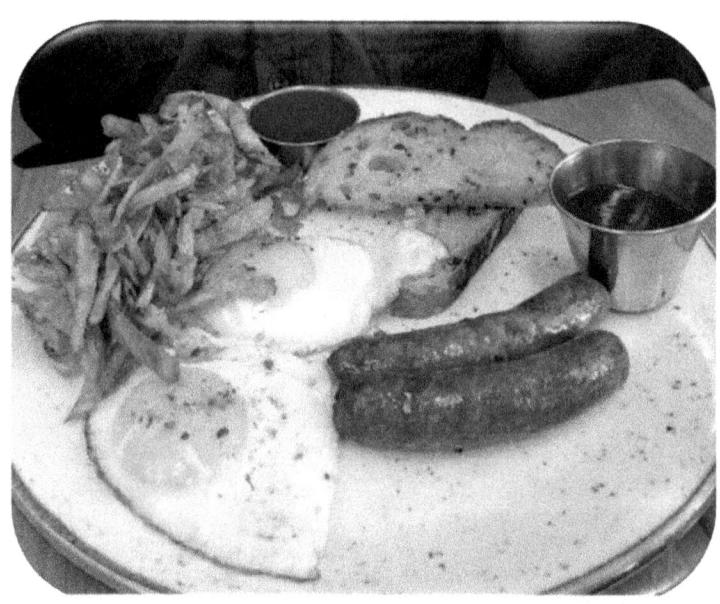

Ingredients:

- 1 pound of lean ground turkey
- 1 tsp of fennel seed
- ¼ tsp garlic powder
- ¼ tsp onion powder
- ¼ tsp salt
- 2 tbsp of vegetable oil
- Pepper

Directions:

Combine all the Ingredientsapart from the vegetable oil in a mixing bowl.

Form into long and flat (around 4 inch-long) patties. Heat the vegetable oil in a medium frying pan.

Add 3-4 patties at a time and cook for approx. 3 minutes on each side. Repeat until you cook all patties. Serve warm.

Nutrition	Calories	Fat	Carbs	Protein	Sodium	Phosphorus	Potassium
	174	12g	9g	12g	123mg	78mg	89mg

4. Blueberry Smoothie Bowl

Preparation Time: 1 minutes | Cooking Time: 1 minutes | Servings: 1

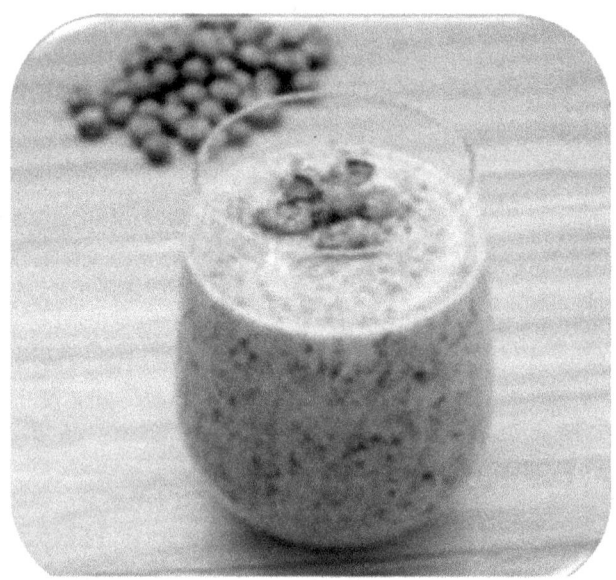

Ingredients:

- ½ cup of frozen blueberries
- ½ cup of vanilla flavored almond milk
- 1 tbsp of agave syrup
- 1 tsp of chia seeds

Directions:

Combine everything except for the chia seeds in the blender until smooth. You should end up with a thick smoothie paste.

Transfer into a cereal bowl and top with chia seeds on top.

Nutrition	Calories	Fat	Carbs	Protein	Sodium	Phosphorus	Potassium
	278	6g	39g	1.5g	76mg	59mg	229mg

5. Egg White and Pepper Omelets

Preparation Time: 2 minutes | *Cooking Time:* 5 minutes | *Servings:* 1-2

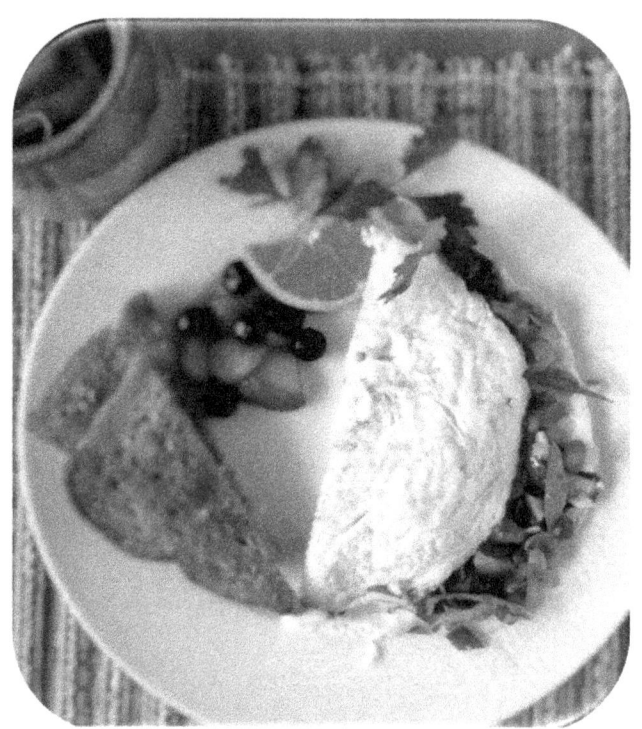

Ingredients:

- 4 egg whites, lightly beaten
- 1 red bell pepper, diced
- 1 tsp of paprika
- 2 tbsp. of olive oil
- ½ tsp of salt
- Pepper

Directions:

In a shallow pan (around 8 inches), heat the olive oil and sauté the bell peppers until softened.

Add the egg whites and the paprika and fold the edges into the fluid center with a spatula and let omelet cook until eggs are fully opaque and solid.

Season with salt and pepper.

Nutrition	Calories	Fat	Carbs	Protein	Sodium	Phosphorus	Potassium
	164	6g	3.9g	9.3g	767mg	202mg	193mg

6. Chicken Egg Rolls

Preparation Time: 10 minutes | *Cooking Time:* 12 minutes | *Servings:* 9

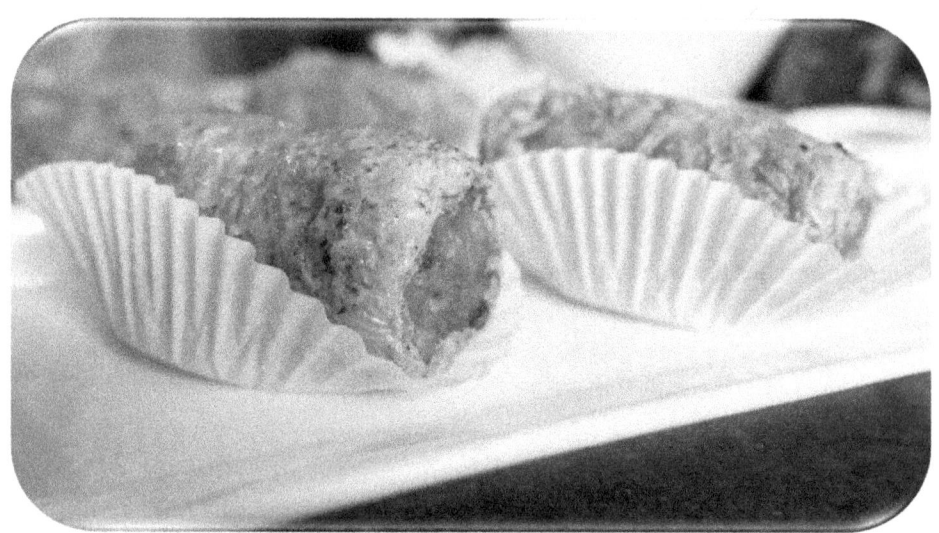

Ingredients:

- 1 lb. cooked chicken, diced
- 1/2 lb. bean sprouts
- 1/2 lb. cabbage, shredded
- 1 cup onion, chopped
- 2 tablespoons olive oil
- 1 tablespoon low sodium soy sauce
- 1 garlic clove, minced
- 20 egg roll wrappers
- Oil for frying

Directions:

Add everything to a suitable bowl except for the roll wrappers. Mix these Ingredientswell to prepare the filling then marinate for 30 minutes.

Place the roll wrappers on the working surface and divide the prepared filling on them. Fold the roll wrappers as per the package instructions and keep them aside.

Add oil to a deep wok and heat it to 350°F. Deep the egg rolls until golden brown on all sides, then transfer the egg rolls to a plate lined with a paper towel to absorb all the excess oil. Serve warm.

Nutrition	Calories	Fat	Carbs	Protein	Sodium	Phosphorus	Potassium
	212	4g	29g	14.3g	329mg	361mg	173mg

7. **Pork Bread Casserole**

Preparation Time: *20 minutes* | ***Cooking Time***: *55 minutes* | ***Servings***: *8*

Ingredients:

- 2 tablespoons butter
- 1 lb. pork sausage
- 1 yellow onion, chopped
- 18 slices white bread, cut into cubes
- 2 ½ cups sharp Cheddar cheese, grated
- 1/2 cup fresh parsley, chopped
- 6 large eggs
- 2 cups half-and-half cream
- 1 teaspoon garlic powder
- 1/4 teaspoon black pepper

Directions:

Switch on your gas oven and preheat it at 325°F. Layer a 9x9 inches casserole dish with bread cubes.

Set a suitable-sized skillet over medium-high heat then crumb the sausage in it.

Cook the sausage until golden brown, then keep it aside. Blend the eggs with the remaining Ingredientsin a blender until smooth.

Stir in the sausage and spread this mixture over the bread pieces.

Bake the bread casserole for 55 minutes approximately in the preheated oven. Slice and serve.

Nutrition	Calories	Fat	Carbs	Protein	Sodium	Phosphorus	Potassium
	366	15g	15g	17.3g	467mg	501mg	231mg

8. Salmon Bagel Toast

Preparation Time: 10 minutes | *Cooking Time*: 5 minutes | *Servings*: 2

Ingredients:

- 1 plain bagel, cut in half
- 2 tablespoons cream cheese
- 1/3 cup English cucumber, thinly sliced
- 3 oz. smoked salmon, sliced
- 3 rings red onion
- 1/2 teaspoon capers, drained

Directions:

Toast each half of the bagel in a skillet until golden brown.

Cover one of the toasted halves with cream cheese. Set the cucumber, salmon, and capers on top of each bagel half.

Nutrition	Calories	Fat	Carbs	Protein	Sodium	Phosphorus	Potassium
	223	6g	27g	13.9g	1137mg	79mg	151mg

Lunch Recipes

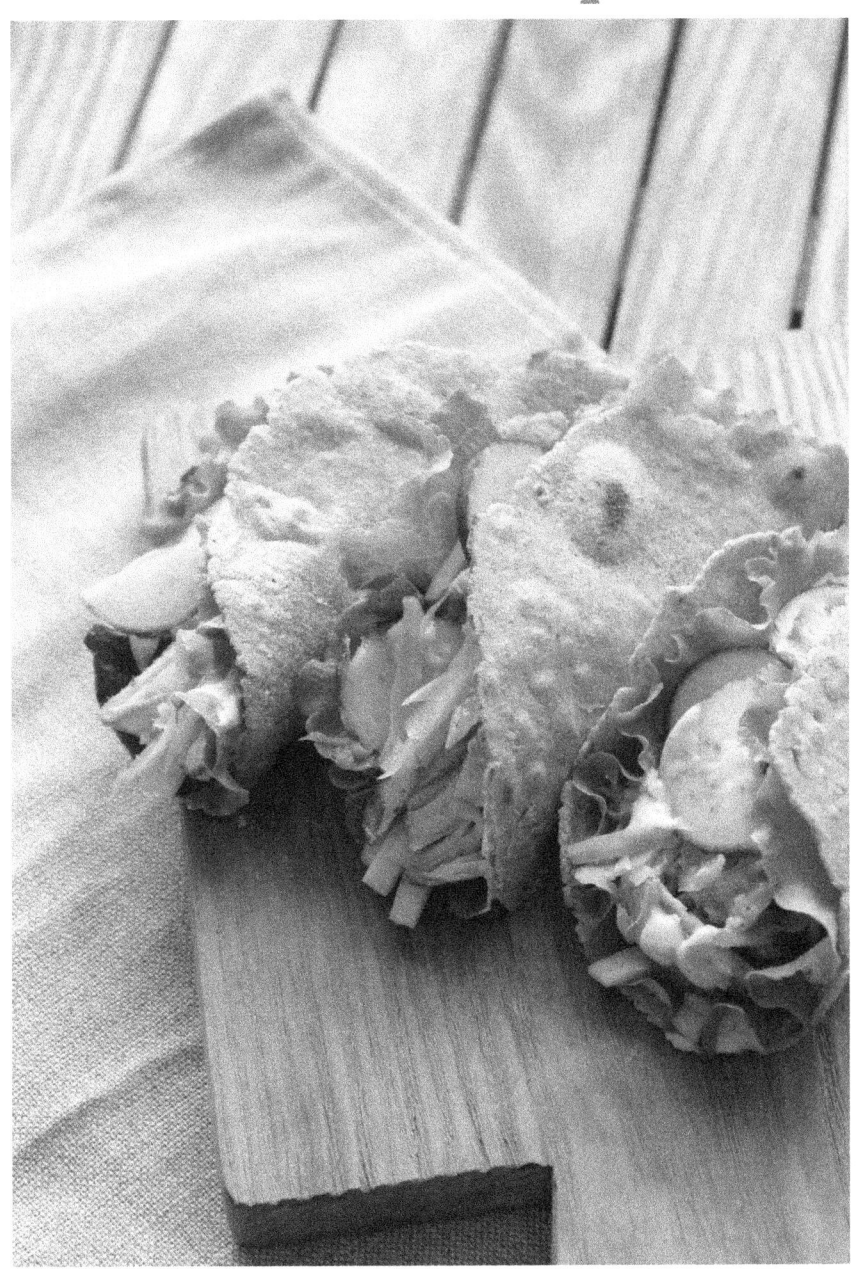

9. Authentic Shrimp Wraps

Preparation Time: 20 minutes | Cooking Time: 15 minutes | Servings: 4

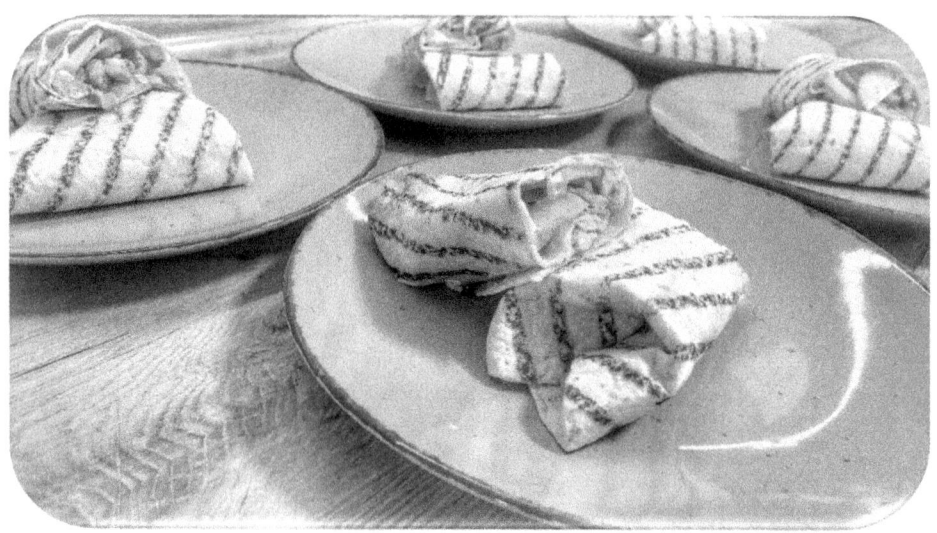

Ingredients:

- For Filling:
- 1 tbsp. of olive oil
- 1 minced garlic clove
- 1 seeded and chopped medium red bell pepper
- ½ pound of peeled, deveined and chopped medium shrimp
- Pinch of salt
- Freshly ground black pepper, to taste
- For Wraps:
- 4 large lettuce leaves

Directions:

In a large skillet, heat oil on medium heat. Add garlic and sauté for about 30 seconds.

Add bell pepper and cook for about 2-3 minutes.

Add shrimp and seasoning and cook for about 2-3 minutes. Remove from heat and cool slightly.

Divide shrimp mixture over lettuce leaves evenly. Serve immediately.

Nutrition	Calories	Fat	Carbs	Protein	Sodium	Phosphorus	Potassium
	97	4.3g	2g	12.3g	169mg	51mg	81mg

10. Loveable Tortillas

Preparation Time: 60 minutes | *Cooking Time:* 15 minutes | *Servings:* 8

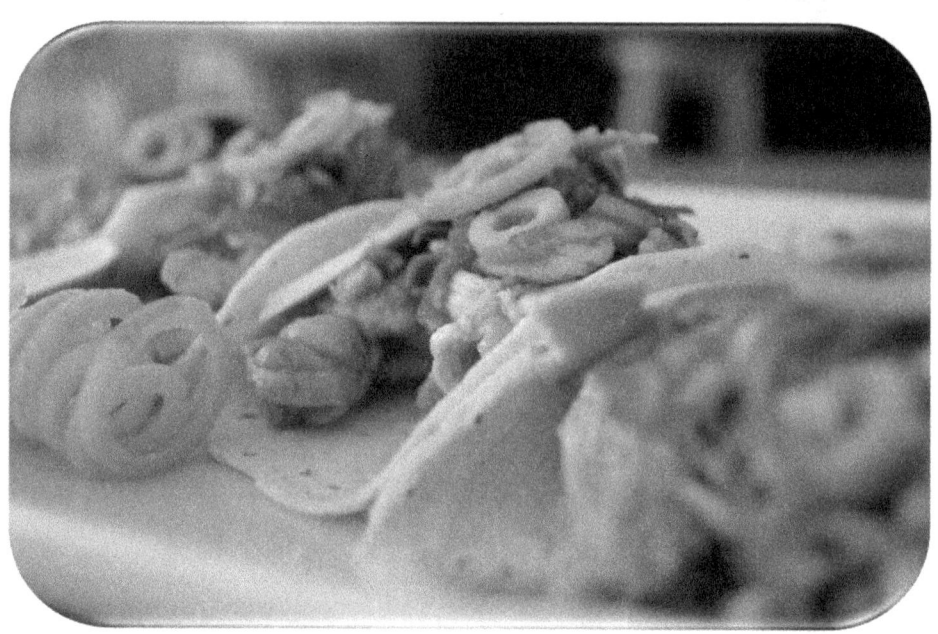

Ingredients:

- ½ cup of low-sodium mayonnaise
- 1 finely minced garlic clove
- 8-ounce of chopped unsalted cooked chicken
- ½ of seeded and chopped red bell pepper
- ½ of seeded and chopped green bell pepper
- 1 chopped red onion
- 4 (6-ounce) warmed corn tortillas

Directions:

In a bowl, mix together mayonnaise and garlic.

In another bowl, mix together chicken and vegetables. Arrange the tortillas onto smooth surface.

Spread mayonnaise mixture over each tortilla evenly. Place chicken mixture over ¼ of each tortilla.

Fold the outside edges inward and roll up like a burrito. Secure each tortilla with toothpicks to secure the filling. Cut each tortilla in half and serve.

Nutrition	Calories	Fat	Carbs	Protein	Sodium	Phosphorus	Potassium
	297	8.2g	44g	13.3g	171mg	99mg	269mg

11. Elegant Veggie Tortillas

Preparation Time: 30 minutes | Cooking Time: 15 minutes | Servings: 9

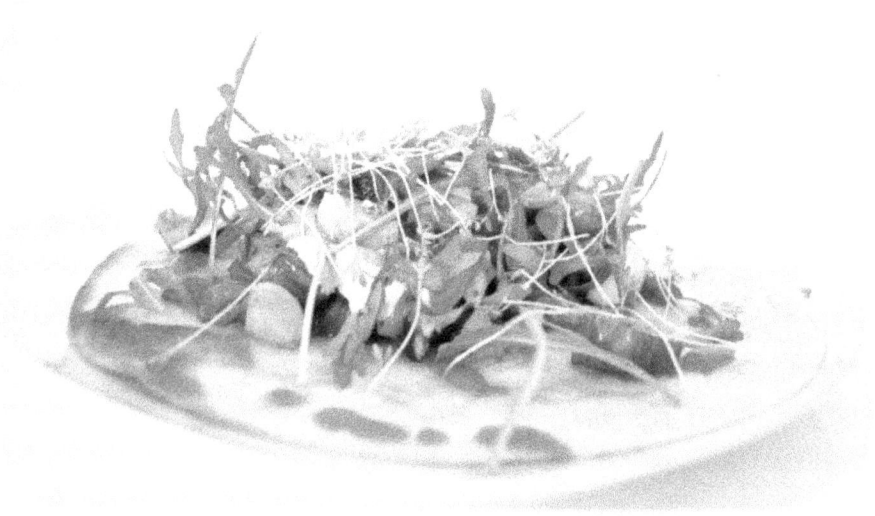

Ingredients:

- 1½ cups of chopped broccoli florets
- 1½ cups of chopped cauliflower florets
- 1 tbsp. of water
- 2 tsp. of canola oil
- 1½ cups of chopped onion
- 1 minced garlic clove
- 2 tbsp. of finely chopped fresh parsley
- 1 cup of low-cholesterol liquid egg substitute
- black pepper, to taste
- 4 warmed corn tortillas

Directions:

In a microwave bowl, place broccoli, cauliflower and water and microwave, covered for about 3-5 minutes. Remove from microwave and drain any liquid.

In a skillet, heat oil on medium heat. Add onion and sauté for about 4-5 minutes.

Add garlic and sauté for about 1 minute. Stir in broccoli, cauliflower, parsley, egg substitute and black pepper. Reduce the heat to medium-low and simmer for about 10 minutes.

Remove from heat and keep aside to cool slightly, then place broccoli mixture over ¼ of each tortilla. Fold the outside edges inward and roll up like a burrito.

Secure each tortilla with toothpicks to secure the filling. Cut each tortilla in half and serve.

Nutrition	Calories	Fat	Carbs	Protein	Sodium	Phosphorus	Potassium
	217	32g	21g	8.3g	87mg	59mg	289mg

12. Delightful Pizza

Preparation Time: 40 minutes | *Cooking Time*: 15 minutes | *Servings*: 4

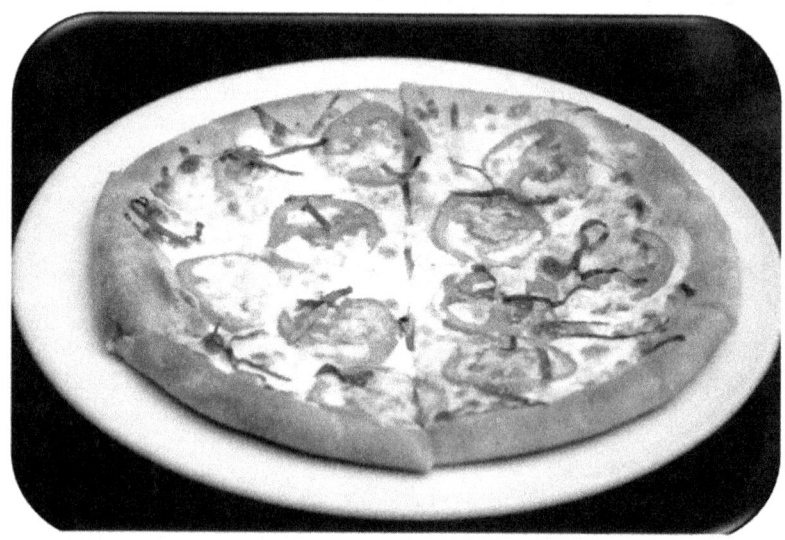

Ingredients:

- 2 pita breads
- 3 tbsp. low-sodium tomato sauce
- 3-ounce of cubed unsalted cooked chicken
- ¼ cup of chopped onion
- 2 tbsp. of crumbled feta cheese

Directions:

Preheat the oven to 350°F. Grease a baking sheet, then arrange the pita breads onto prepared baking sheet.

Spread the barbecue sauce over each pita bread evenly. Top with chicken and onion evenly and sprinkle with cheese. Bake for about 11-13 minutes.

Cut each pizza in half and serve.

Nutrition	Calories	Fat	Carbs	Protein	Sodium	Phosphorus	Potassium
	133	2.2g	18.2g	9.3g	271mg	59mg	29mg

13. Winner Kabobs

Preparation Time: 50 minutes | *Cooking Time:* 15 minutes | *Servings:* 6

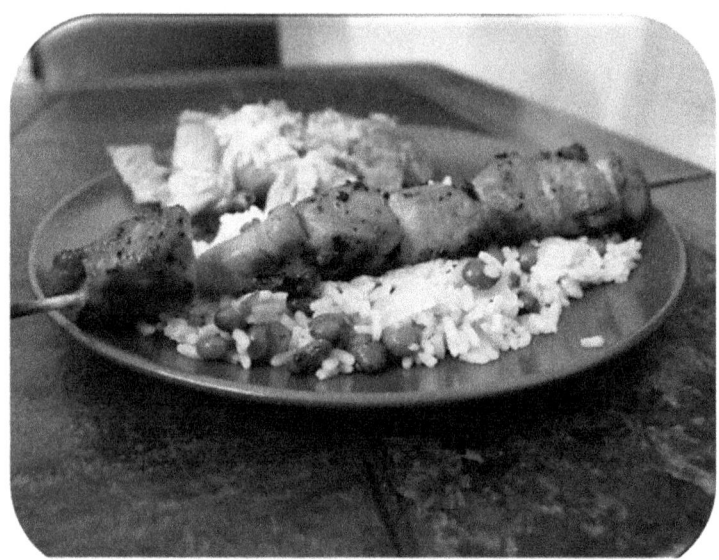

Ingredients:

- 1 pound of cubed skinless, boneless chicken breast
- 1 seeded and cut into 1-inch pieces medium red bell pepper
- 1 seeded and cut into 1-inch pieces medium green bell pepper
- 20-ounce of cut into 1-inch pieces pineapple
- 1 cut into 1-inch pieces red onion
- 1/3 cup of low-sodium barbecue sauce
- Freshly ground black pepper, to taste

Directions:

Preheat the outdoor grill to medium-high heat. Lightly, grease the grill grate.

Thread chicken, bell peppers, pineapple and onion onto pre-soaked 6 wooden skewers.

Coat all the ingredients with ½ of barbecue sauce and sprinkle with black pepper.

Place the skewers in prepared baking sheet in a single layer. Grill the skewers for about 9-10 minutes, flipping occasionally.

Remove from grill and immediately, coat with remaining barbecue sauce. Serve immediately.

Nutrition	Calories	Fat	Carbs	Protein	Sodium	Phosphorus	Potassium
	182	3g	21g	18.3g	185mg	21mg	234mg

14. Tempting Burgers

Preparation Time: 20 minutes | *Cooking Time:* 15 minutes | *Servings:* 6

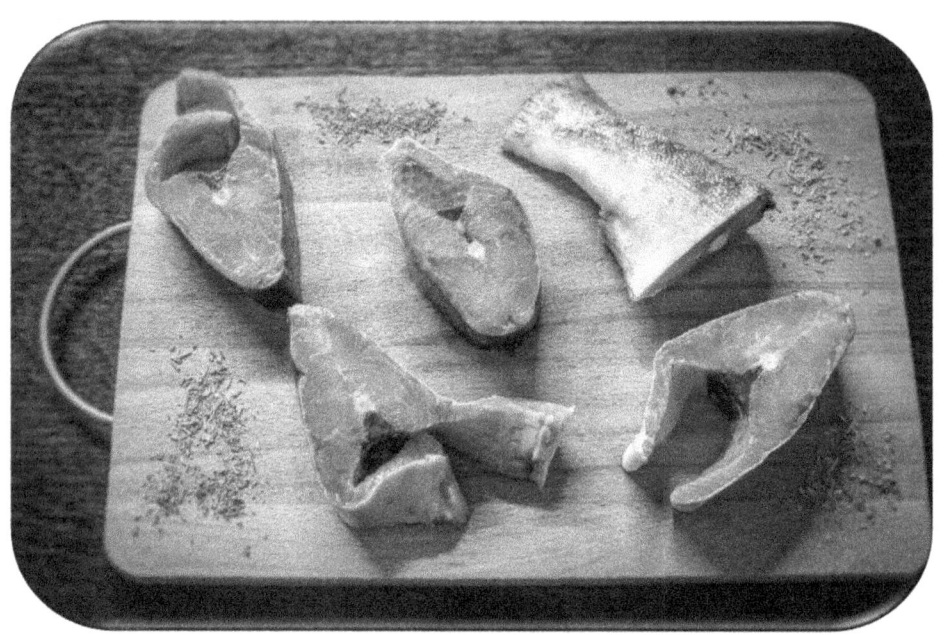

Ingredients:

- 12-ounce of finely chopped unsalted cooked salmon
- ½ cup of minced onion
- 1 minced garlic clove
- 2 tbsp. of chopped fresh parsley
- 1 large egg
- ½ tsp. of paprika
- Ground black pepper, to taste
- 2 tbsp. of olive oil
- 3 cups torn lettuce

Directions:

Preheat the oven to 350°F. Line a baking sheet with parchment paper. In a large bowl, add all ingredients, except oil and mix until well combined.

Make equal sized 12 patties from mixture. Place patties onto prepared baking dish in a single layer.

Bake for about 12-15 minutes. Now, in a large skillet, heat oil on high heat.

Remove salmon burgers from oven and transfer into skillet. Cook for about 1 minute per side.

Divide lettuce in serving plates evenly. Place 2 patties in each plate and serve.

Nutrition	Calories	Fat	Carbs	Protein	Sodium	Phosphorus	Potassium
	136	9g	2.1g	12.3g	31mg	59mg	295mg

15. Caraway Cabbage And Rice

Preparation Time: 5 minutes | *Cooking Time*: 10 minutes | *Servings*: 2

Ingredients:

- 1 cup of rice, cooked
- ¼ cup mandarin oranges
- 1 tablespoon white onion, chopped
- 1 cup cabbage, shredded
- ½ teaspoon caraway seed
- 1 tablespoon Worcestershire sauce
- ¼ cup water

Directions:

Take a frying pan, grease it with oil, place it over medium heat, add onion and cabbage and cook for 5 minutes until cabbage leaves wilted.

Stir in caraway seeds, Worcestershire sauce, and water, continue cooking for 3 minutes, add oranges and stir until rice until well combined.

Serve straight away.

Nutrition	Calories	Fat	Carbs	Protein	Sodium	Phosphorus	Potassium
	142	0g	31g	3g	71mg	59mg	205mg

16. Gratin Pasta With Watercress And Chicken

Preparation Time: 10 minutes | *Cooking Time*: 50 minutes | *Servings*: 4

Ingredients:

- 2 cups pasta shells, cooked
- 1 cup chicken, shredded and cooked
- 1 white onion, peeled and chopped
- 1 cup fresh watercress
- 1 teaspoon minced garlic
- ¼ teaspoon ground black pepper
- 1 tablespoon olive oil
- ½ cup Parmesan cheese, grated
- 1 2/3 cup béchamel sauce

Directions:

Take a medium-sized skillet pan, place it over medium heat, add oil and when hot, add onion and garlic, and cook for 4 minutes until saluted.

Then stir in chicken and watercress until mixed and continue cooking for 3 minutes until leaves of watercress have wilted.

Add pasta, pour in half of the béchamel sauce, mix until coated, and spoon the mixture into a greased baking dish.

Cover pasta with remaining béchamel sauce, sprinkle cheese on top and bake for 40 minutes until cheese has melts and pasta is bubbling.

Serve straight away.

Nutrition	Calories	Fat	Carbs	Protein	Sodium	Phosphorus	Potassium
	345	13g	38g	19g	101mg	39mg	20mg

Dinner Recipes

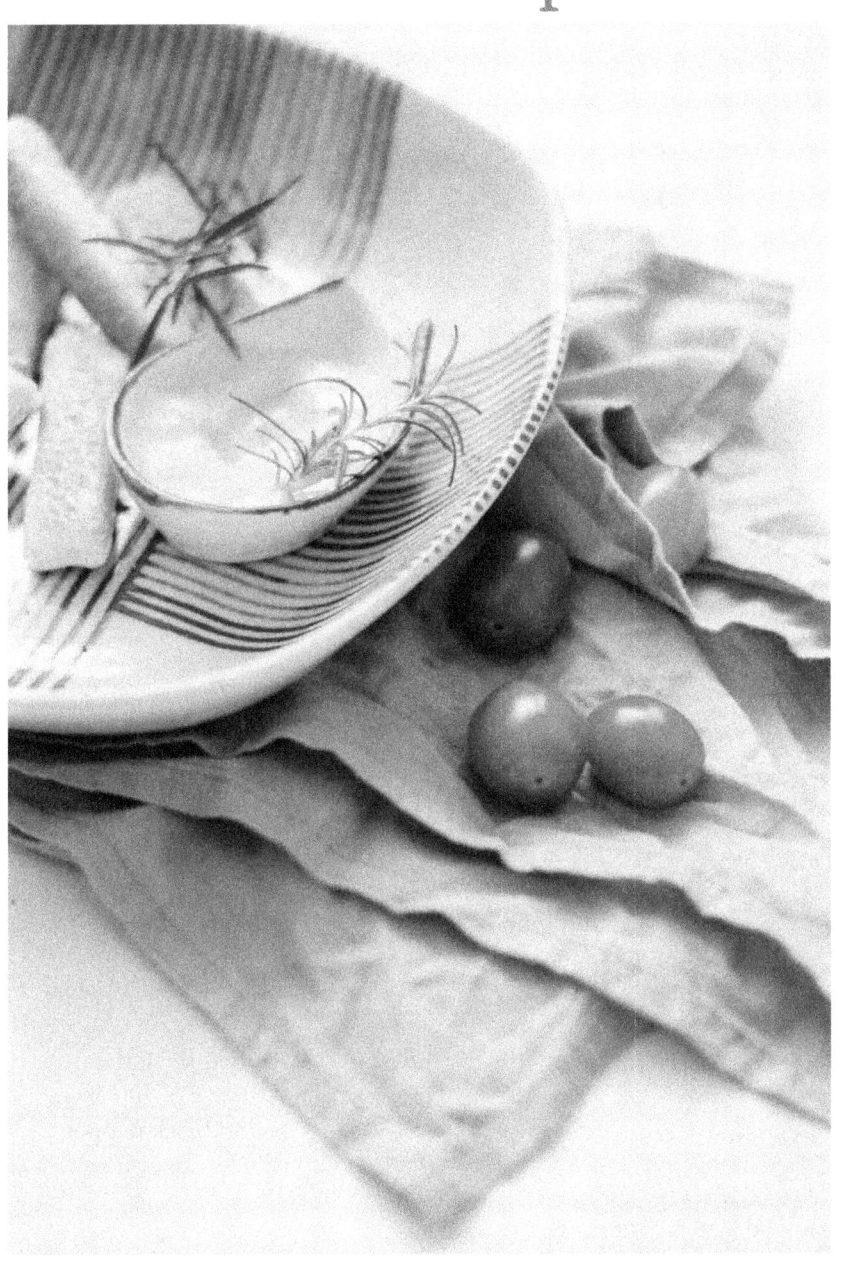

17. Ground Beef And Rice Soup

Preparation Time: 15 minutes | *Cooking Time*: 40 minutes | *Servings*: 4

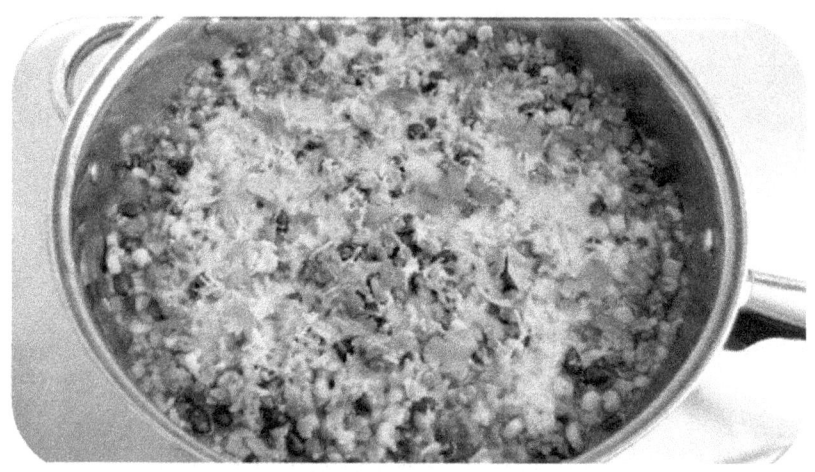

Ingredients:

- Extra-lean ground beef – ½ pound
- Sweet onion – ½, chopped
- Minced garlic – 1 tsp.
- Water – 2 cups
- 1 cup low-sodium beef broth
- Long-grain white rice – ½ cup, uncooked
- Celery stalk – 1, chopped
- Fresh green beans – ½ cup, cut into – 1-inch pieces
- Chopped fresh thyme – 1 tsp.
- Ground black pepper

Directions:

Sauté the ground beef in a saucepan for 6 minutes or until the beef is completely browned.

Drain off the excess fat and add the onion and garlic to the saucepan.

Sauté the vegetables for about 3 minutes, or until they are softened. Add the celery, rice, beef broth, and water.

Bring the soup to a boil, reduce the heat to low and simmer for 30 minutes or until the rice is tender.

Add the green beans and thyme and simmer for 3 minutes. Remove the soup from the heat and season with pepper.

Nutrition	Calories	Fat	Carbs	Protein	Sodium	Phosphorus	Potassium
	154	7g	14g	9g	133mg	201mg	217mg

18. Persian Chicken

Preparation Time: 10 minutes | *Cooking Time:* 20 minutes | *Servings:* 5

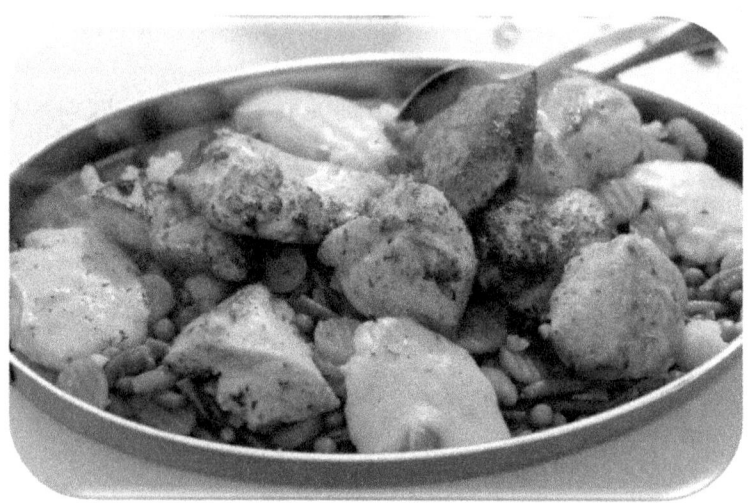

Ingredients:

- Sweet onion – ½, chopped
- Lemon juice – ¼ cup
- Dried oregano – 1 Tbsp.
- Minced garlic – 1 tsp.
- Sweet paprika – 1 tsp.
- Ground cumin – ½ tsp.
- Olive oil – ½ cup
- Boneless, skinless chicken thighs – 5

Directions:

Put the cumin, paprika, garlic, oregano, lemon juice, and onion in a food processor and pulse to mix the ingredients.

Keep the motor running and add the olive oil until the mixture is smooth.

Place the chicken thighs in a large sealable freezer bag and pour the marinade into the bag. Seal the bag and place in the refrigerator, turning the bag twice, for 2 hours.

Remove the thighs from the marinade and discard the extra marinade. Preheat the barbecue to medium.

Grill the chicken for about 20 minutes, turning once, until it reaches 165°F.

Nutrition	Calories	Fat	Carbs	Protein	Sodium	Phosphorus	Potassium
	321	21g	3g	22g	86mg	71mg	137mg

19. Eggplant and Red Pepper Soup

Preparation Time: 20 minutes | *Cooking Time*: 40 minutes | *Servings*: 6

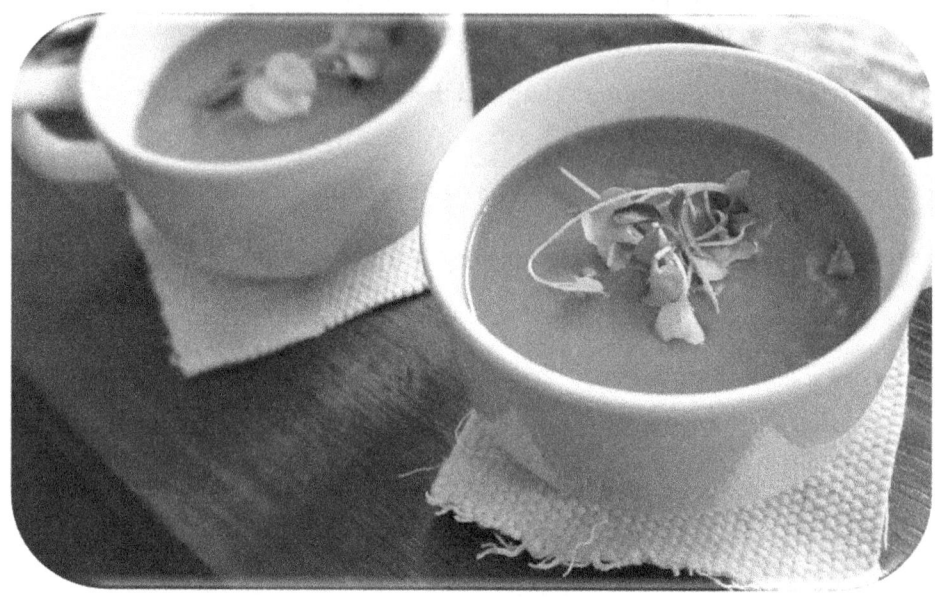

Ingredients:

- Sweet onion – 1 small, cut into quarters
- Red bell peppers – 2, halved
- Cubed eggplant – 2 cups
- Garlic – 2 cloves, crushed
- Olive oil – 1 Tbsp.
- Chicken stock – 1 cup
- Water
- Chopped fresh basil – ¼ cup
- Ground black pepper to taste

Directions:

Preheat the oven to 350°F. Put the onions, red peppers, eggplant, and garlic in a baking dish. Drizzle the vegetables with the olive oil.

Roast the vegetables for 30 minutes or until they are slightly charred and soft, the cool the vegetables slightly and remove the skin from the peppers.

Puree the vegetables with a hand mixer (with the chicken stock). Transfer the soup to a medium pot and add enough water to reach the desired thickness.

Heat the soup to a simmer and add the basil. Season with pepper and serve.

Nutrition	Calories	Fat	Carbs	Protein	Sodium	Phosphorus	Potassium
	61	2g	9g	2g	98mg	110mg	144mg

20. Seafood Casserole

Preparation Time: 20 minutes | *Cooking Time:* 45 minutes | *Servings:* 6

Ingredients:

- Eggplant – 2 cups, peeled and diced into 1-inch pieces
- Butter, for greasing the baking dish
- Olive oil – 1 tbsp.
- Sweet onion – ½, chopped
- Minced garlic - 1 tsp.
- Celery stalk – 1, chopped
- Red bell pepper – ½, boiled and chopped
- Freshly squeezed lemon juice – 3 Tbsps.
- Hot sauce – 1 tsp.
- Creole seasoning mix – ¼ tsp.
- White rice – ½ cup, uncooked
- Egg – 1 large
- Cooked shrimp – 4 ounces
- Queen crab meat – 6 ounces

Directions:

Preheat the oven to 350°F. Boil the eggplant in a saucepan for 5 minutes, then drain and set aside.

Grease a 9-by-13-inch baking dish with butter and set aside.

Heat the olive oil in a large skillet over medium heat. Sauté the garlic, onion, celery, and bell pepper for 4 minutes or until tender.

Add the sautéed vegetables to the eggplant, along with the lemon juice, hot sauce, seasoning, rice, and egg.

Stir to combine. Fold in the shrimp and crab meat. Spoon the casserole mixture into the casserole dish, patting down the top.

Bake for 25 to 30 minutes or until casserole is heated through and rice is tender. Serve warm.

Nutrition	Calories	Fat	Carbs	Protein	Sodium	Phosphorus	Potassium
	118	4g	9g	12g	235mg	102mg	197mg

21. Ground Beef and Rice Soup

Preparation Time: 15 minutes | Cooking Time: 40 minutes | Servings: 6

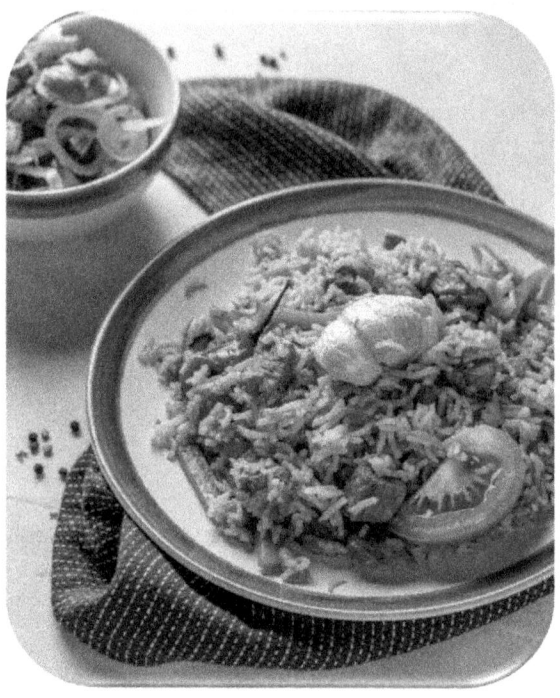

Ingredients:

- Extra-lean ground beef – ½ pound
- Small sweet onion – ½, chopped
- Minced garlic – 1 tsp
- Water – 2 cups
- Low-sodium beef broth – 1 cup
- Long-grain white rice – ½ cup, uncooked
- Celery stalk – 1, chopped
- Fresh green beans – ½ cup, cut into – 1-inch pieces
- Chopped fresh thyme – 1 tsp
- Ground black pepper

Directions:

Sauté the ground beef in a saucepan for 6 minutes or until the beef is completely browned. Drain off the excess fat and add the onion and garlic to the saucepan.

Sauté the vegetables for about 3 minutes, or until they are softened. Add the celery, rice, beef broth, and water.

Bring the soup to a boil, reduce the heat to low and simmer for 30 minutes or until the rice is tender.

Add the green beans and thyme and simmer for 3 minutes. Remove the soup from the heat and season with pepper.

Nutrition	Calories	Fat	Carbs	Protein	Sodium	Phosphorus	Potassium
	154	7g	14g	9g	178mg	76mg	179mg

22. Couscous Burgers

Preparation Time: 20 minutes | *Cooking Time:* 10 minutes | *Servings:* 4

Ingredients:

- Canned chickpeas – ½ cup, rinsed and drained
- Chopped fresh cilantro – 2 Tbsps
- Chopped fresh parsley
- Lemon juice - 1 Tbsp
- Lemon zest – 2 tsps.
- Minced garlic – 1 tsp.
- Cooked couscous – 2 ½ cups
- Eggs – 2 lightly beaten
- Olive oil – 2 Tbsps

Directions:

Put the cilantro, chickpeas, parsley, lemon juice, lemon zest, and garlic in a food processor and pulse until a paste form.

Transfer the chickpea mixture to a bowl and add the eggs and couscous. Mix well.

Chill the mixture in the refrigerator for 1 hour. Form the couscous mixture into 4 patties.

Heat olive oil in a skillet. Place the patties in the skillet, 2 at a time, gently pressing them down with a spatula.

Cook for 5 minutes or until golden and flip the patties over.

Cook the other side for 5 minutes and transfer the cooked burgers to a plate covered with a paper towel.

Repeat with the remaining 2 burgers.

Nutrition	Calories	Fat	Carbs	Protein	Sodium	Phosphorus	Potassium
	242	10g	29g	9g	43mg	108mg	167mg

23. Baked Flounder

Preparation Time: 20 minutes | Cooking Time: 5 minutes | Servings: 4

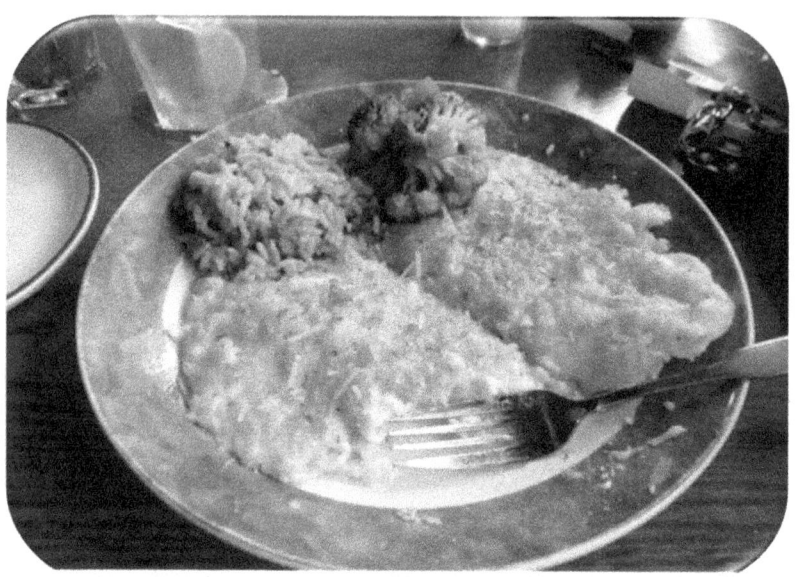

Ingredients:

- Homemade mayonnaise – ¼ cup
- Juice of 1 lime
- Zest of 1 lime
- Chopped fresh cilantro – ½ cup
- Flounder fillets – 4 (3-ounce)
- Ground black pepper

Directions:

Preheat the oven to 400°F. In a bowl, stir together the cilantro, lime juice, lime zest, and mayonnaise.

Place 4 pieces of foil, about 8 by 8 inches square, on a clean work surface.

Place a flounder fillet in the center of each square. Top the fillets evenly with the mayonnaise mixture. Season the flounder with pepper.

Fold the sides of the foil over the fish, creating a snug packet, and place the foil packets on a baking sheet.

Bake the fish for 4 to 5 minutes. Unfold the packets and serve.

Nutrition	Calories	Fat	Carbs	Protein	Sodium	Phosphorus	Potassium
	92	4g	2g	12g	267mg	209mg	137mg

24. Spicy Chicken

Preparation Time: 12 minutes | *Cooking Time:* 25 minutes | *Servings:* 6

Ingredients:

- 1 pounds boneless skinless chicken breasts cut into 1 inch pieces
- 1/3 cup cornstarch
- 1/3 cup buffalo hot sauce
- 1/2 cup brown sugar
- 1/4 cup sliced green onions
- 2 eggs beaten
- 3 tbsp vegetable oil
- 1 tbsp rice vinegar
- 1/4 tbsp red pepper flakes or more to taste
- salt and pepper to taste

Directions:

Preheat the oven to 350°F. Coat a pan with cooking spray and place the chicken pieces on a plate, then season with salt and pepper to taste.

Sprinkle the cornstarch over the chicken and toss to coat evenly.

Dip each piece of chicken into the beaten eggs. Heat the oil over high heat in a large pan.

Place the chicken in a single layer and cook for 5 minutes on each side or until golden brown. You may have to work in batches.

Place the chicken pieces in a single layer in the pan. In a small bowl, whisk together the buffalo sauce, brown sugar, rice vinegar and red pepper flakes.

Pour the sauce over the chicken. Bake for 35 minutes, stirring once halfway through to coat the chicken with the sauce.

Top with green onions and serve.

Nutrition	Calories	Fat	Carbs	Protein	Sodium	Phosphorus	Potassium
	321	17g	5g	25g	101mg	109mg	237mg

Snacks & Sides Recipes

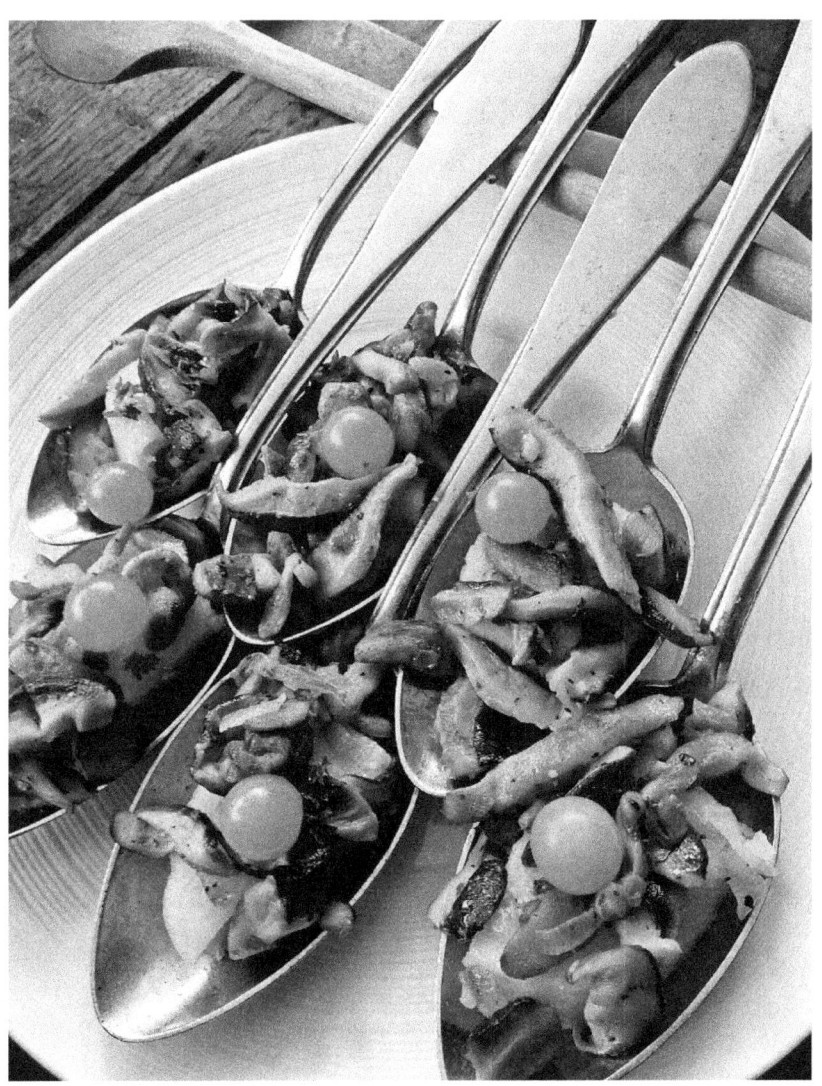

25. Eggplant Sandwich

Preparation Time: *30 minutes* | *Cooking Time*: *30 minutes* | *Servings*: *2*

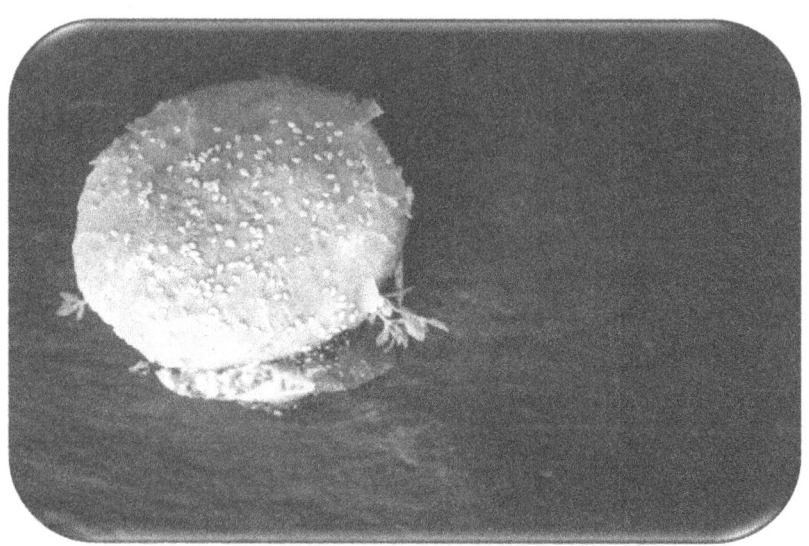

Ingredients:

- 1 eggplant, sliced
- 2 teaspoons parsley, dried
- Salt and pepper to the taste
- ½ cup vegan breadcrumbs
- ½ teaspoon Italian seasoning
- ½ teaspoon garlic powder
- ½ teaspoon onion powder
- 2 tablespoons almond milk
- 4 vegan bread slices
- Cooking spray
- ½ cup avocado mayo
- ¾ cup tomato sauce
- A handful basil, chopped

Directions:

Season eggplant slices with salt and pepper, leave aside for 30 minutes and then pat dry them well.

In a bowl, mix parsley with breadcrumbs, Italian seasoning, onion and garlic powder, salt and black pepper and stir. In another bowl, mix milk with vegan mayo and also stir well.

Brush eggplant slices with mayo mix, dip them in breadcrumbs mix, place them on a lined baking sheet, spray with cooking

oil, introduce baking sheet in your air fryer's basket and cook them at 400°F for 15 minutes, flipping them halfway.

Brush each bread slice with olive oil and arrange 2 of them on a working surface.

Add baked eggplant slices, spread tomato sauce and basil and top with the other bread slices, greased side down. Divide between plates and serve.

Nutrition	Calories	Fat	Carbs	Protein	Sodium	Phosphorus	Potassium
	324	16g	19g	12g	104mg	104mg	201mg

26. Date and Blueberry Muffins

Preparation Time: 20 minutes | *Cooking Time:* 30 minutes | *Servings:* 9

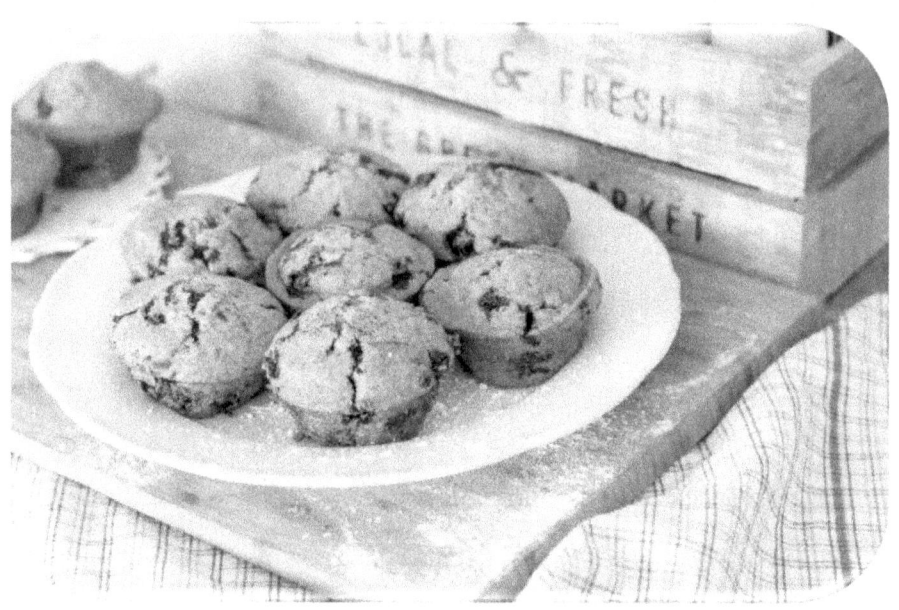

Ingredients:

- 2 tablespoons flax meal
- 6 tablespoons water
- 1 cup almond flour
- 1 cup coconut flour
- 2 teaspoons baking soda
- 1 teaspoon sea salt
- 2 tablespoons mixed spice
- 1 cup dates, pitted
- 2 cups canned pumpkin
- 1 teaspoon lemon juice
- ¼ cup coconut oil
- 5 ounces frozen blueberries
- ¾ cup zucchini, grated
- ¾ cup chopped walnuts

Directions:

Preheat oven to 350° F. Line 12 muffin cups with paper liners.

Mix together the flax meal and water and leave for a few minutes until it becomes a gel-like consistency.

Mix almond flour, coconut flour, baking soda, sea salt and mixed spice in large bowl. Set aside.

In a food processor, pulse together the pitted dates, pumpkin and lemon juice together with the flax water and coconut oil, then mix the pumpkin mixture into the dry ingredients. Mix well.

Gently stir in the blueberries, grated zucchini and walnuts. Divide the mixture evenly between the prepared muffin cups.

Bake for about 30 minutes. If the muffins are too gooey, after this time, leave for a few minutes longer.

Nutrition	Calories	Fat	Carbs	Protein	Sodium	Phosphorus	Potassium
	211	12g	23g	5g	109mg	104mg	212mg

27. Cranberry and Lemon Cookies

Preparation Time: 20 minutes | *Cooking Time:* 15 minutes | *Servings:* 12

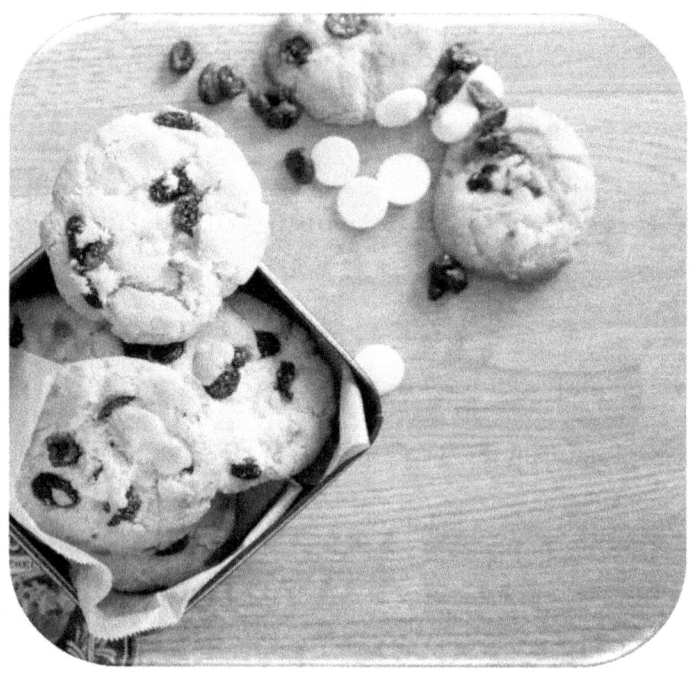

Ingredients:

- ½ cup coconut milk
- 1 tablespoon ground flaxseed
- 1¼ cups brown organic superfine sugar
- ½ cup apple sauce
- ¼ cup vegetable oil
- 1 tablespoon fresh lemon juice
- 1½ teaspoons lemon zest
- 2 teaspoons vanilla extract
- 1¼ cups unbleached general-purpose flour
- 1 cup whole wheat flour
- 1 teaspoon baking soda ½ teaspoon salt
- 1 cup dried cranberries
- 1 cup chopped walnuts

Directions:

Pre-heat the oven to 350°F. Prepare 2 cookie sheets with parchment paper.

Warm the coconut milk and stir in the flaxseed. Leave to one side for it to gel. In a large bowl, stir together all of the wet Ingredients with the sugar. Stir in the gelled flax seed.

In another bowl sift together the flours, baking soda and salt.

Add the flour mix to the wet ingredients a little at a time until fully combined.

When a dough has formed stir in the nuts and cranberries. Using a spoon form 2-inch round cookies on the prepared sheets.

Bake for 12 – 15 minutes until a nice golden brown.

Remove from the oven and leave to rest on the cookie sheet for about 5 minutes. Place on a cooling rack. Serve, eat and enjoy!

Nutrition	Calories	Fat	Carbs	Protein	Sodium	Phosphorus	Potassium
	332	14g	47.8g	5g	170mg	153mg	202mg

28. No Bake Oat Cookies

Preparation Time: *30 minutes* | ***Cooking Time***: *0 minutes* | ***Servings***: *24*

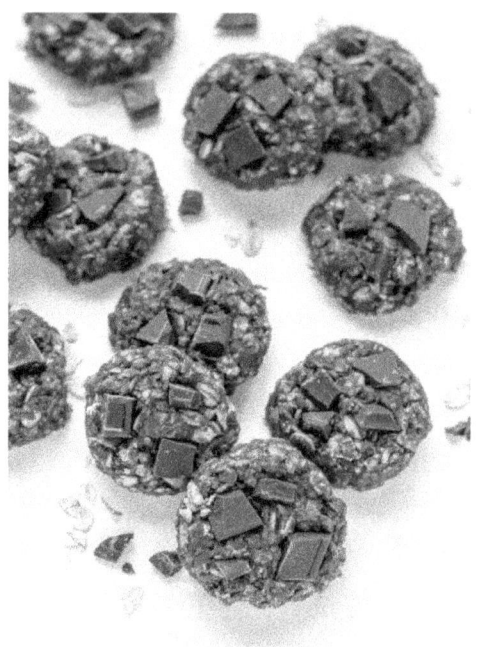

Ingredients:

- ½ cup plain soymilk
- 1¾ cups sugar
- ½ cup Vegan butter
- 1 teaspoon vanilla extract
- 3½ cups quick cooking oats
- ¼ cup unsweetened cocoa powder
- ½ cup smooth or crunchy peanut butter

Directions:

In a small pot combine the milk, butter, sugar, peanut butter and vanilla and cook until smooth and creamy

In a large bowl combine the oats and cocoa powder. Pour the warm milk mixture over the oats and stir until all the ingredients have combined.

Place dollops of mixture onto a waxed paper lined cookie sheet and let cool for about half an hour.

Nutrition	Calories	Fat	Carbs	Protein	Sodium	Phosphorus	Potassium
	171	7g	25.5g	3.3g	96mg	97mg	101mg

29. Chocolate Coconut Quinoa Slices

Preparation Time: 10 minutes | *Cooking Time*: 25 minutes | *Servings*: 12

Ingredients:

- ¾ cup quinoa
- ½ cup dried chopped dates
- 3 tablespoons maple syrup
- 2 tablespoons olive oil
- 2 tablespoons ground flaxseed
- ½ teaspoon almond extract
- ¼ teaspoon salt
- ½ cup chocolate protein powder
- ½ cup whole wheat flour
- ¼ cup Vegan chocolate chips
- ¼ cup shredded coconut Water

Directions:

Pre-heat the oven to 350°F. Prepare an 8 x 8 ovenproof baking dish. Grease lightly with oil. Rinse the quinoa in cold water and leave to soak for about 10 minutes.

Drain the quinoa. Place 1 cup of water in a small saucepan bring to the boil. Add the quinoa and simmer over a low heat for about 12 minutes. Cool.

In a food processor combine the cooked quinoa, dates, maple syrup, olive oil, flaxseed, almond extract and salt.

Process until fairly smooth. In a separate bowl stir together the chocolate protein powder, flour chocolate chips and coconut.

Fold the dry mixture into the wet mixture with a flat spatula or knife.

Press into the prepared baking dish. Even out the top. Bake for about 25 minutes, until firm.

Cool and then slice into bars. Store in an airtight container for about a week or freeze up to 3 months.

Nutrition	Calories	Fat	Carbs	Protein	Sodium	Phosphorus	Potassium
	160	5g	22.4g	9g	38mg	78mg	92mg

30. Pineapple Raspberry Parfaits

Preparation Time: 6 minutes | *Cooking Time*: 0 minutes | *Servings*: 2

Ingredients:

- ½ pint fresh raspberries
- 1 ½ cup fresh or frozen pineapple chunks
- 2 8oz containers non-fat peach yogurt

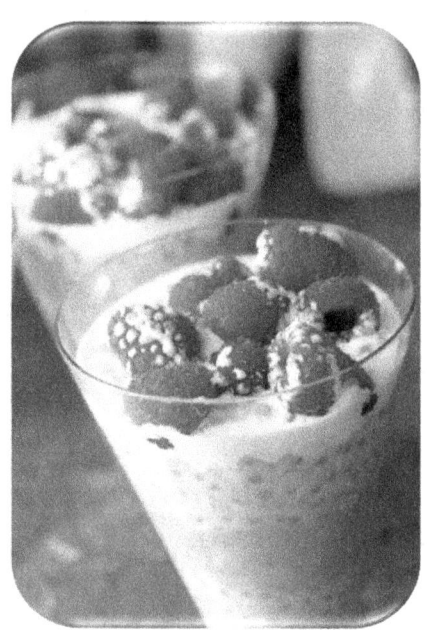

Directions:

In a parfait glass, layer the yogurt, raspberries and pineapples alternately. Chill inside the refrigerator. Serve chilled.

Nutrition	Calories	Fat	Carbs	Protein	Sodium	Phosphorus	Potassium
	319	1g	60g	22g	85mg	93mg	472mg

Desserts Recipes

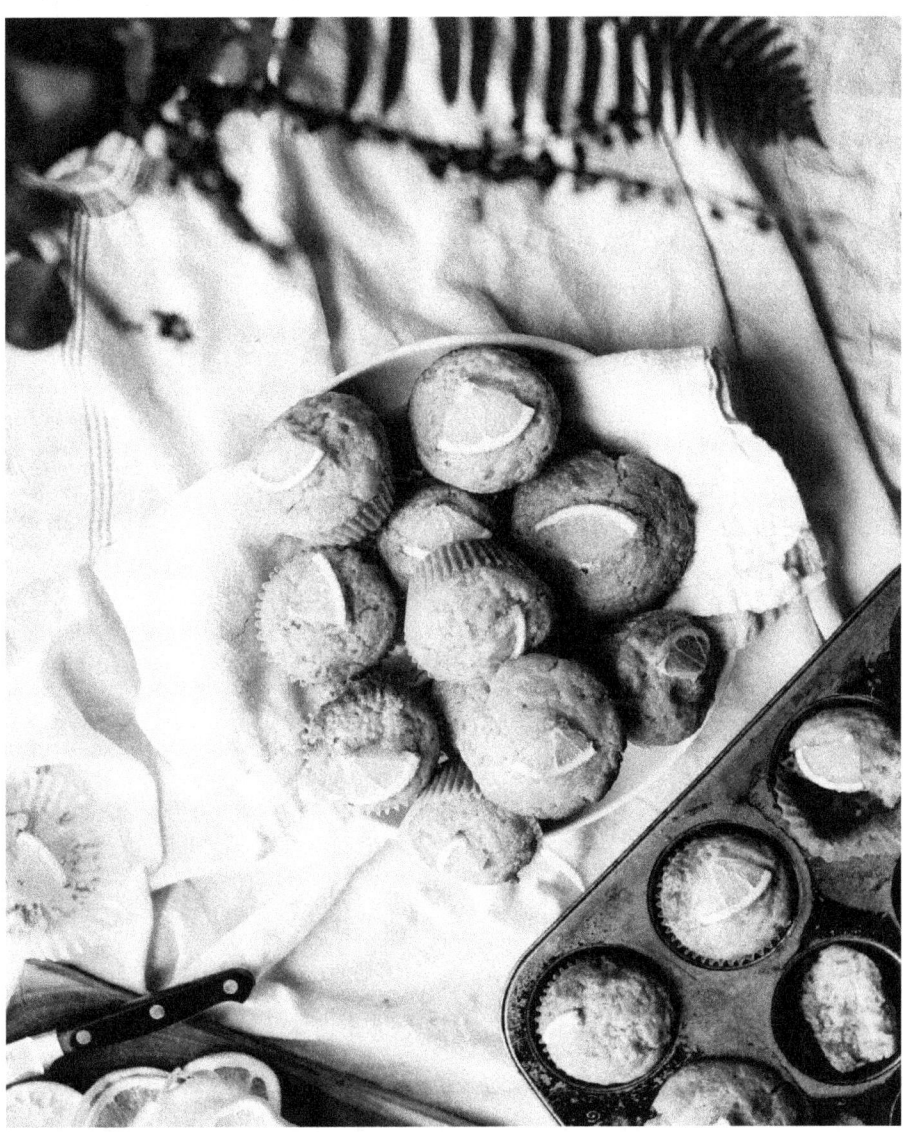

31. Simple Berry Sorbet

Preparation Time: 5 minutes | *Cooking Time*: 5 minutes | *Servings*: 1

Ingredients:

- 1/2 cup fresh raspberries
- 1/2 cup fresh strawberries
- 5 drops liquid stevia
- 1 tsp fresh lemon juice

Directions:

Add all ingredients into the blender and blend until smooth.

Pour into the air-tight container and place it in the freezer for 3-4 hours.

Serve chilled and enjoy.

Nutrition	Calories	Fat	Carbs	Protein	Sodium	Phosphorus	Potassium
	55	0.8g	12g	1.3g	82mg	74mg	142mg

32. Chocolate Mousse

Preparation Time: 5 minutes | *Cooking Time:* 5 minutes | *Servings:* 4

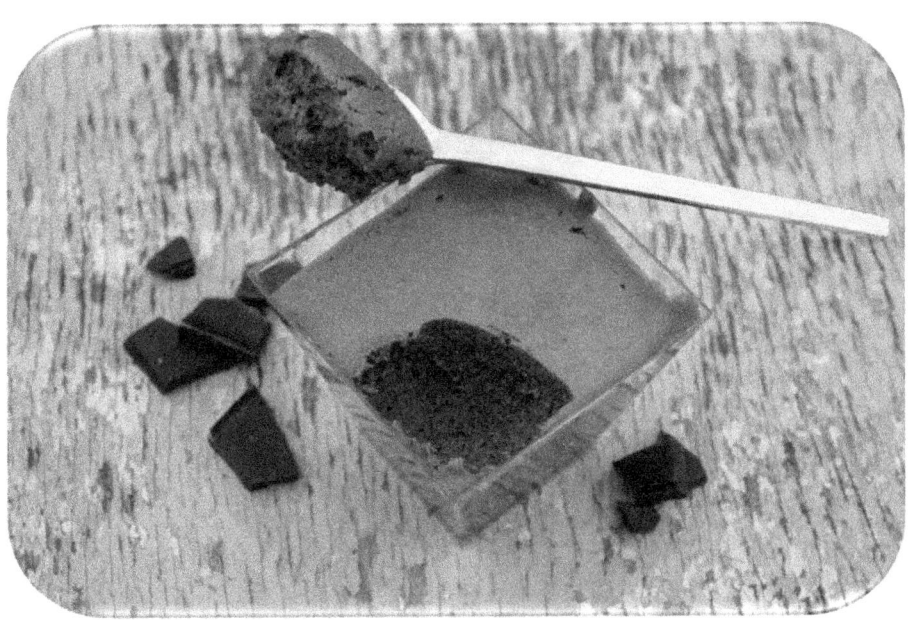

Ingredients:

- 1/2 cup unsweetened cocoa powder
- 1/2 tsp vanilla
- 1 1/4 cup heavy cream
- 4 oz cream cheese
- 8 drops liquid stevia

Directions:

Add all ingredients into the blender and blend until smooth and creamy.

Pour mixture into the serving bowls and place in the refrigerator for 1-2 hours.

Serve and enjoy.

Nutrition	Calories	Fat	Carbs	Protein	Sodium	Phosphorus	Potassium
	255	24g	6g	5.1g	144mg	93mg	182mg

33. Keto Brownie

Preparation Time: 10 minutes | *Cooking Time*: 20 minutes | *Servings*: 4

Ingredients:

- 2 tbsp unsweetened cocoa powder
- 1/2 cup almond butter, melted
- 1 cup banana, overripe & mashed
- 1 scoop vanilla protein powder
- 1/2 tsp vanilla

Directions:

Preheat the oven to 350° F. Line baking dish with parchment paper and set aside.

Add all ingredients into the blender and blend until smooth. Pour batter into the prepared dish and bake for 20 minutes. Slice and serve.

Nutrition	Calories	Fat	Carbs	Protein	Sodium	Phosphorus	Potassium
	81	2g	10g	7g	77mg	44mg	47mg

34. Smooth Coffee Mousse

Preparation Time: 5 minutes | *Cooking Time*: 5 minutes | *Servings*: 8

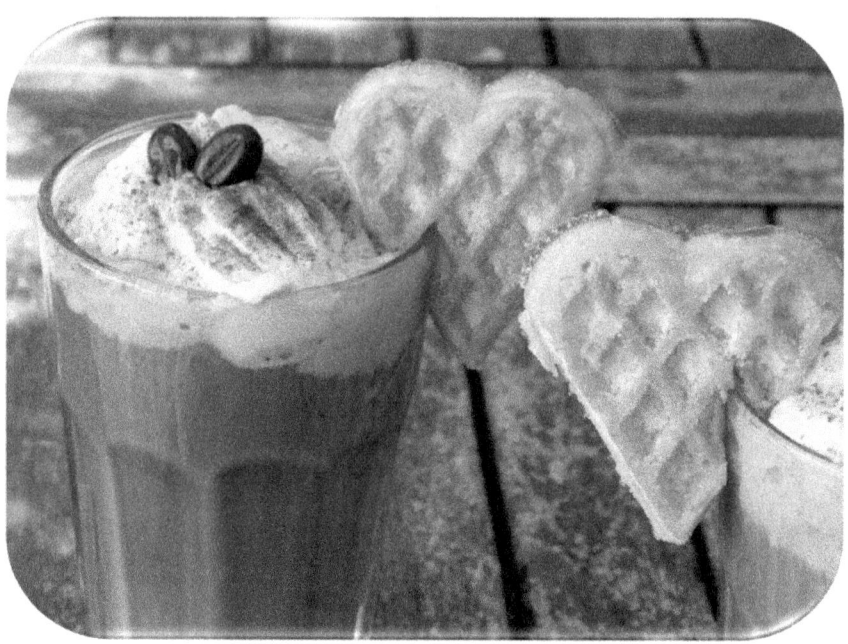

Ingredients:

- 1 cup heavy whipping cream
- 1/2 cup almond milk
- 4 tbsp brewed coffee
- 15 oz cream cheese, softened
- 15 drops liquid stevia
- 1 tsp vanilla

Directions:

Add coffee and cream cheese in a blender and blend until smooth. Add stevia, vanilla, and almond milk and blend until smooth.

Add heavy cream and blend until thickened. Pour into the serving bowls and place in refrigerator 1-2 hours. Serve and enjoy.

Nutrition	Calories	Fat	Carbs	Protein	Sodium	Phosphorus	Potassium
	241	24g	2g	4.4g	177mg	98mg	241mg

35. Almond Bites

Preparation Time: 10 minutes | *Cooking Time:* 10 minutes | *Servings:* 12

Ingredients:

- 1/2 cup almond meal
- 2 tbsp coconut butter
- 4 dates, pitted and chopped
- 1/4 cup unsweetened chocolate chips
- 1 1/2 tsp vanilla

Directions:

Add dates in the food processor and process for 30 seconds.

Add remaining Ingredients except chocolate chips and process until combined. Add chocolate chips and process for 15 seconds.

Make small balls from mixture and place on a baking tray. Place in refrigerator for 1-2 hours. Serve and enjoy

Nutrition	Calories	Fat	Carbs	Protein	Sodium	Phosphorus	Potassium
	53	3.8g	4.2g	1.1g	102mg	47mg	102mg

36. Chocolate Cookies

Preparation Time: 10 minutes | *Cooking Time*: 10 minutes | *Servings*: 18

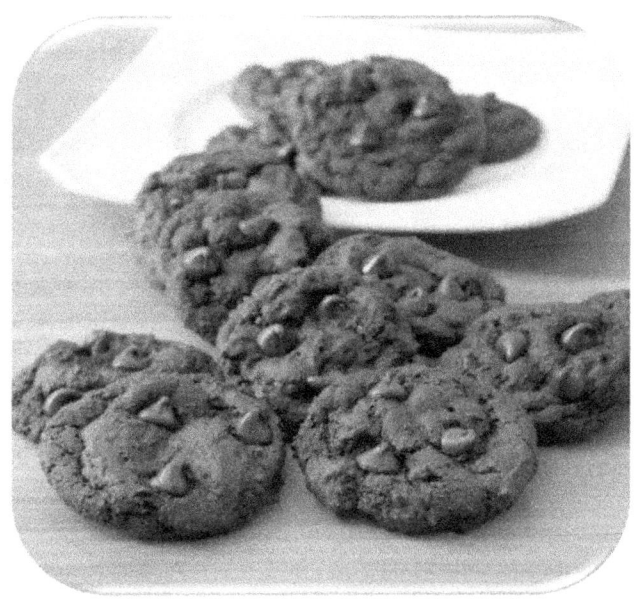

Ingredients:

- 2 eggs, lightly beaten
- 3 tbsp butter
- 3 tbsp cocoa powder
- 1 1/2 cups almond flour
- 1 tsp vanilla
- 1/4 cup Swerve
- 3 oz chocolate, chopped
- Pinch of salt

Directions:

Add chocolate, butter, and cocoa powder into the pan and melt over medium-low heat. Remove from heat and set aside.

Add eggs, vanilla, salt, and swerve in a bowl and blend until well combined. Add melted chocolate mixture into the egg mixture and mix well.

Add almond flour and mix until well combined. Place in refrigerator for 1 hour.

Preheat the oven to 325 °F. Line baking tray with parchment paper and spray with cooking spray.

Scoop out batter onto a baking tray and bake for 10 minutes. Serve and enjoy.

Nutrition	Calories	Fat	Carbs	Protein	Sodium	Phosphorus	Potassium
	66	5g	4.9g	2g	73mg	73mg	72mg

37. Chocolate Muffins

Preparation Time: 10 minutes | *Cooking Time*: 30 minutes | *Servings*: 10

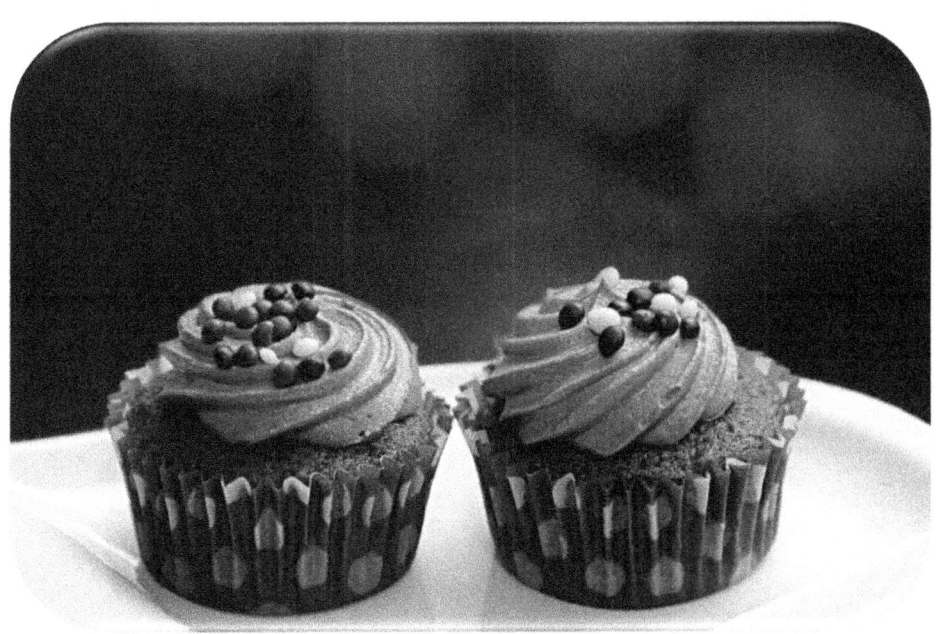

Ingredients:

- 2 eggs, lightly beaten
- 1/2 cup cream
- 1/2 tsp vanilla
- 1 cup almond flour
- 1 tbsp baking powder, gluten-free
- 4 tbsp Swerve
- 1/2 cup cocoa powder
- Pinch of salt

Directions:

Preheat the oven to 375°F. Spray a muffin tray with cooking spray and set aside.

In a mixing bowl, mix together almond flour, baking powder, swerve, cocoa powder, and salt. In a separate bowl, beat eggs with cream, and vanilla.

Pour egg mixture into the almond flour mixture and mix well.

Pour batter into the prepared muffin tray and bake in preheated oven for 30 minutes. Serve and enjoy.

Nutrition	Calories	Fat	Carbs	Protein	Sodium	Phosphorus	Potassium
	101	8g	6.7g	4.5g	46mg	47mg	114mg

Smoothies & Drinks

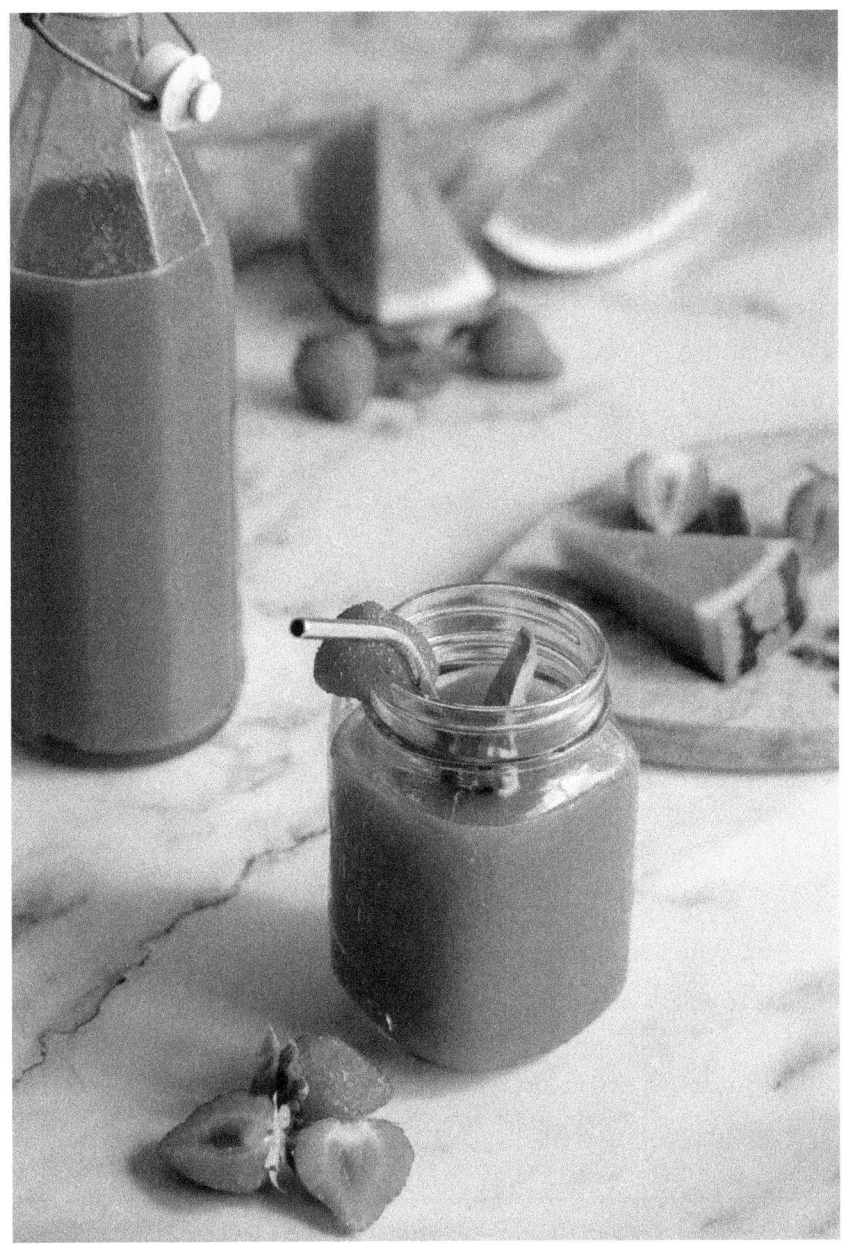

38. Dark Turnip Greens Smoothie

Preparation Time: 10 minutes | *Cooking Time:* 3 minutes | *Servings:* 2

Ingredients:

- 1 cup of raw turnip greens
- 1 1/2 cup of almond milk
- 1 Tbsp of almond butter
- 1/2 cup of water
- 1/2 tsp of cocoa powder, unsweetened
- 1 Tbsp of dark chocolate chips
- 1/4 tsp of cinnamon
- A pinch of salt
- 1/2 cup of crushed ice

Directions:

Rinse and clean turnip greens from any dirt. Place the turnip greens in your blender along with all other ingredients.

Blend it for 45 - 60 seconds or until done; smooth and creamy. Serve with or without crushed ice.

Nutrition	Calories	Fat	Carbs	Protein	Sodium	Phosphorus	Potassium
	131	10g	5g	4g	28mg	0.1mg	19mg

39. Butter Pecan and Coconut Smoothie

Preparation Time: 5 minutes *Cooking Time*: 2 minutes *Servings*: 2

Ingredients:

- 1 cup coconut milk, canned
- 1 scoop Butter Pecan powdered creamer
- 2 cups fresh spinach leaves, chopped
- 1/2 banana frozen or fresh
- 2 Tbsp stevia granulated sweetener to taste
- 1/2 cup water
- 1 cup ice cubes crushed

Directions:

Place ingredients from the list above in your high-speed blender.

Blend for 35 - 50 seconds or until all ingredients combined well. Add less or more crushed ice. Drink and enjoy!

Nutrition	Calories	Fat	Carbs	Protein	Sodium	Phosphorus	Potassium
	268	26g	7g	4g	71mg	73mg	114mg

40. Fresh Cucumber, Kale and Raspberry Smoothie

Preparation Time: 10 minutes | *Cooking Time*: 3 minutes | *Servings*: 3

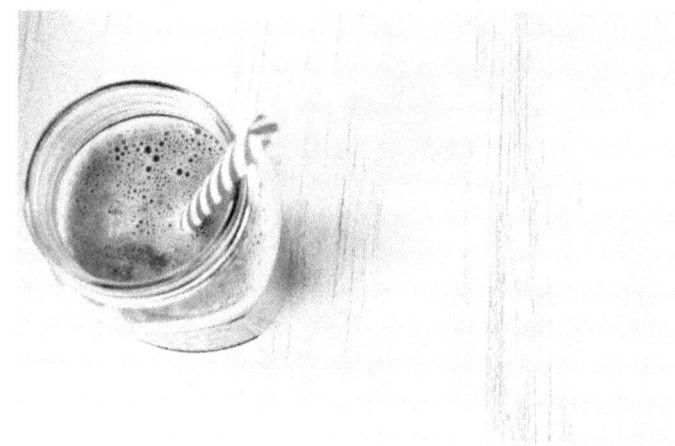

Ingredients:

- 1 1/2 cups of cucumber, peeled
- 1/2 cup raw kale leaves
- 1 1/2 cups fresh raspberries
- 1 cup of almond milk
- 1 cup of water
- Ice cubes crushed
- 2 Tbsp natural sweetener

Directions:

Place all ingredients from the list in a food processor or high-speed blender; blend for 35 - 40 seconds.

Serve into chilled glasses. Add more natural sweeter if you like. Enjoy!

Nutrition	Calories	Fat	Carbs	Protein	Sodium	Phosphorus	Potassium
	70	6g	8g	3g	65mg	13mg	45mg

41. Fresh Lettuce and Cucumber-Lemon Smoothie

Preparation Time: 10 minutes | *Cooking Time:* 3 minutes | *Servings:* 2

Ingredients:

- 2 cups fresh lettuce leaves, chopped (any kind)
- 1 cup of cucumber
- 1 lemon washed and sliced.
- 1/2 avocado
- 2 Tbsp chia seeds
- 1 1/2 cup water or coconut water
- 1/4 cup stevia granulate sweetener (or to taste)

Directions:

Add all ingredients from the list above in the high-speed blender; blend until completely smooth. Pour your smoothie into chilled glasses and enjoy!

Nutrition	Calories	Fat	Carbs	Protein	Sodium	Phosphorus	Potassium
	51	4g	4g	2g	19mg	47mg	101mg

42. Green Coconut Smoothie

Preparation Time: 10 minutes | *Cooking Time*: 3 minutes | *Servings*: 2

Ingredients:

- 1 1/4 cup coconut milk (canned)
- 2 Tbsp chia seeds
- 1 cup of fresh kale leaves
- 1 cup of spinach leaves
- 1 scoop vanilla protein powder
- 1 cup ice cubes
- Granulated stevia sweetener (to taste; optional)
- 1/2 cup water

Directions:

Rinse and clean kale and the spinach leaves from any dirt. Add all Ingredients in your blender. Blend until you get a nice smoothie. Serve into chilled glass.

Nutrition	Calories	Fat	Carbs	Protein	Sodium	Phosphorus	Potassium
	179	18g	5g	4g	19mg	61mg	91mg

43. Instant Coffee Smoothie

Preparation Time: 20 minutes | *Cooking Time:* 7 minutes | *Servings:* 2

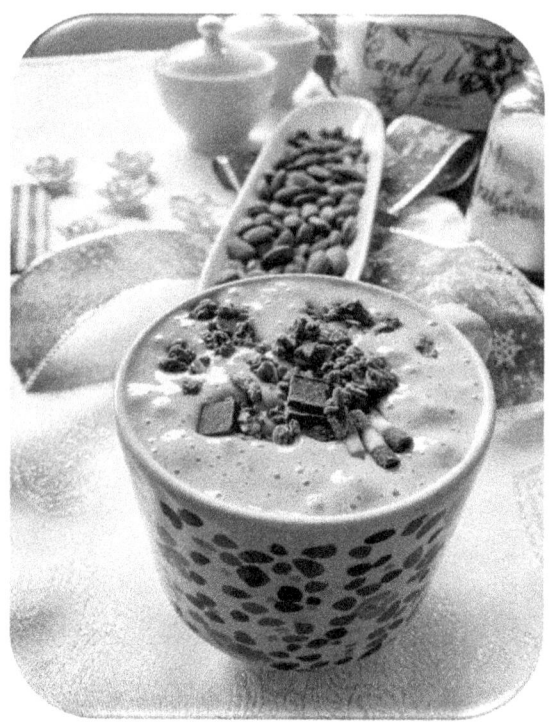

Ingredients:

- 2 cups of instant coffee
- 1 cup almond milk
- 1/4 cup heavy cream
- 2 Tbsp cocoa powder
- 1 Handful of fresh spinach leaves
- 10 drops liquid stevia

Directions:

Make a coffee; set aside. Place all remaining Ingredients in your fast-speed blender; blend for 45 - 60 seconds or until done.

Pour your instant coffee in a blender and continue to blend for further 30 - 45 seconds. Serve immediately.

Nutrition	Calories	Fat	Carbs	Protein	Sodium	Phosphorus	Potassium
	142	14g	6g	5g	46mg	35mg	73mg

44. Keto Blood Sugar Adjuster Smoothie

*Preparation Time: 10 minutes | **Cooking Time**: 3 minutes | **Servings**: 2*

Ingredients:

- 2 cups of green cabbage
- 1/2 avocado
- 1 Tbsp Apple cider vinegar
- Juice of 1 small lemon
- 1 cup of water
- 1 cup of crushed ice cubes For serving

Directions:

Place all ingredients in your high-speed blender or in a food processor and blend until smooth and soft.

Serve in chilled glasses with crushed ice.

Nutrition	Calories	Fat	Carbs	Protein	Sodium	Phosphorus	Potassium
	74	6g	6g	2g	19mg	61mg	13mg

Salads

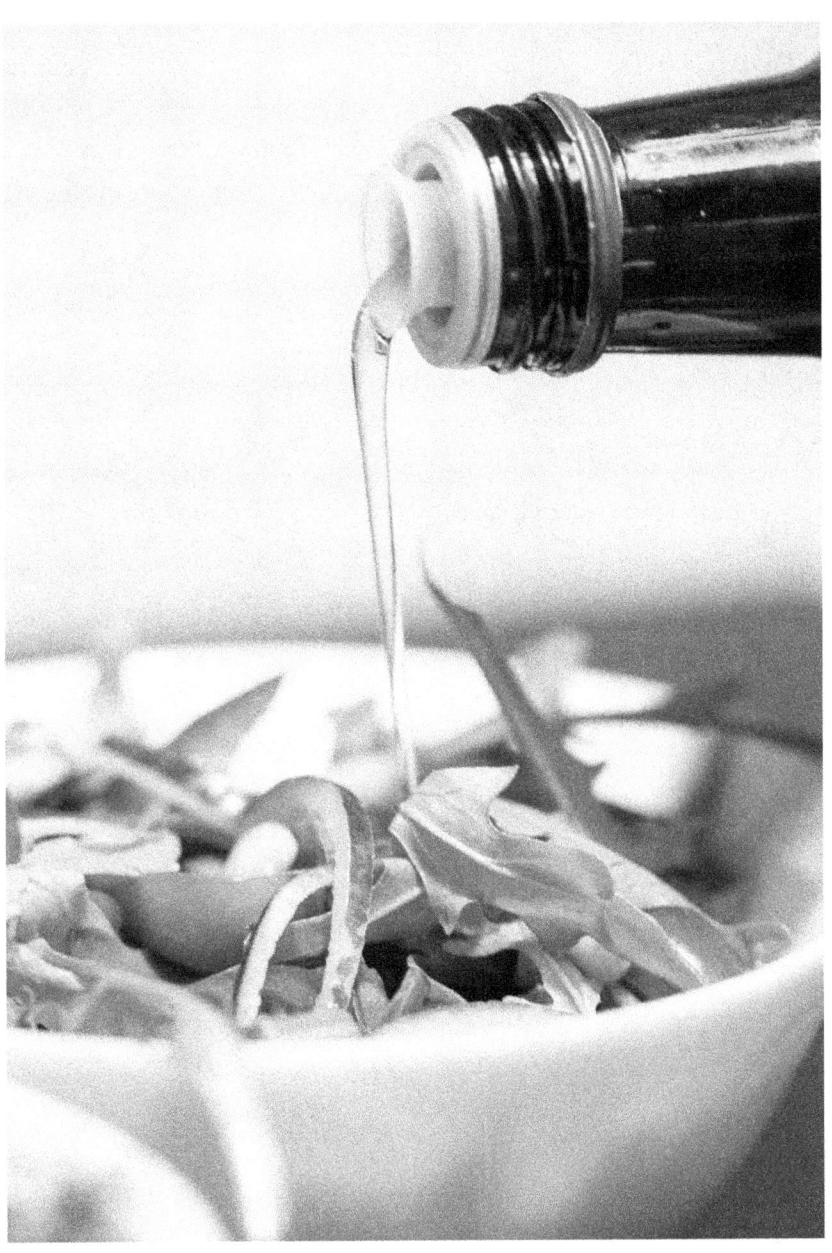

45. Chestnut Noodle Salad

Preparation Time: *10 minutes* | *Cooking Time*: *0 minutes* | *Servings*: *6*

Ingredients:

- 8 cups cabbage, shredded
- 1/2 cup canned chestnuts, sliced
- 6 green onions, chopped
- 1/4 cup olive oil
- 1/4 cup apple cider vinegar
- 3/4 teaspoon stevia
- 1/8 teaspoon black pepper
- 1 cup chow Mein noodles, cooked

Directions:

Take a suitable salad bowl. Start tossing in all the Ingredients:. Mix well and serve.

Nutrition	Calories	Fat	Carbs	Protein	Sodium	Phosphorus	Potassium
	191	13g	6g	4.2g	78mg	188mg	302mg

46. Cranberry Broccoli Salad

Preparation Time: 10 minutes | *Cooking Time*: 0 minutes | *Servings*: 4

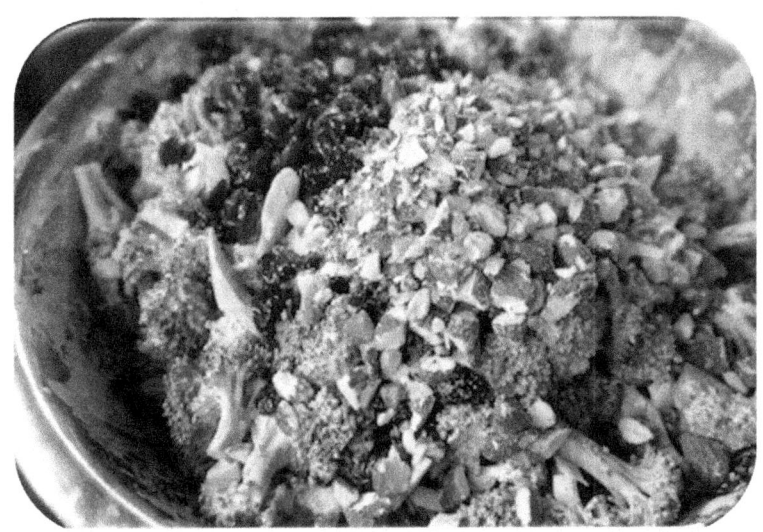

Ingredients:

- 3/4 cup plain Greek yogurt
- 1/4 cup mayonnaise
- 2 tablespoons maple syrup
- 2 tablespoons apple cider vinegar
- 4 cups broccoli florets
- 1 medium apple, chopped
- 1/2 cup red onion, sliced
- 1/4 cup parsley, chopped
- 1/2 cup dried cranberries
- 1/4 cup pecans

Directions:

Put all the salad ingredients into a suitable salad bowl.

Toss them well and refrigerate for 1 hour and serve.

Nutrition	Calories	Fat	Carbs	Protein	Sodium	Phosphorus	Potassium
	252	10g	34g	9.4g	157mg	291mg	480mg

47. Balsamic Beet Salad

Preparation Time: 10 minutes | *Cooking Time:* 0 minutes | *Servings:* 2

Ingredients:

- 1 cucumber, peeled and sliced
- 15 oz. canned low-sodium beets, sliced
- 4 teaspoon balsamic vinegar
- 2 teaspoon sesame oil
- 2 tablespoons Gorgonzola cheese

Directions:

Take a suitable salad bowl.

Start tossing in all the Ingredients:. Mix well and serve.

Nutrition	Calories	Fat	Carbs	Protein	Sodium	Phosphorus	Potassium
	141	8g	16g	5g	426mg	79mg	229mg

48. Shrimp Salad

Preparation Time: 8 minutes | *Cooking Time:* 0 minutes | *Servings:* 4

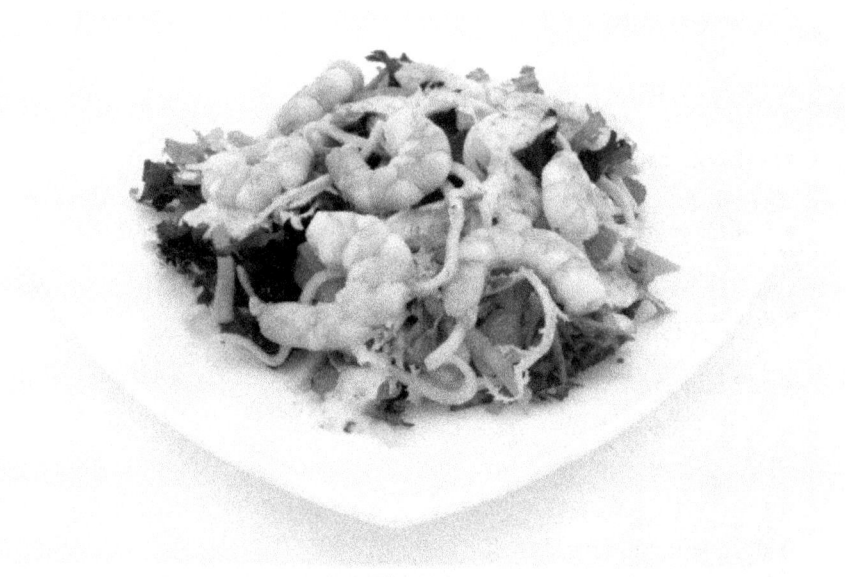

Ingredients:

- 1 lb. shrimp, boiled and chopped
- 1 hardboiled egg, chopped
- 1 tablespoon celery, chopped
- 1 tablespoon green pepper, chopped
- 1 tablespoon onion, chopped
- 2 tablespoons mayonnaise
- 1 teaspoon lemon juice
- ½ teaspoon chili powder
- ⅛ teaspoon hot sauce
- ½ teaspoon dry mustard
- Lettuce, chopped or shredded

Directions:

Take a suitable salad bowl. Start tossing in all the ingredients. Mix well and serve.

Nutrition	Calories	Fat	Carbs	Protein	Sodium	Phosphorus	Potassium
	184	5.7g	4.3g	27.5g	381mg	249mg	233mg

49. Chicken Pomegranate Salad

Preparation Time: 10 minutes | *Cooking Time*: 0 minutes | *Servings*: 6

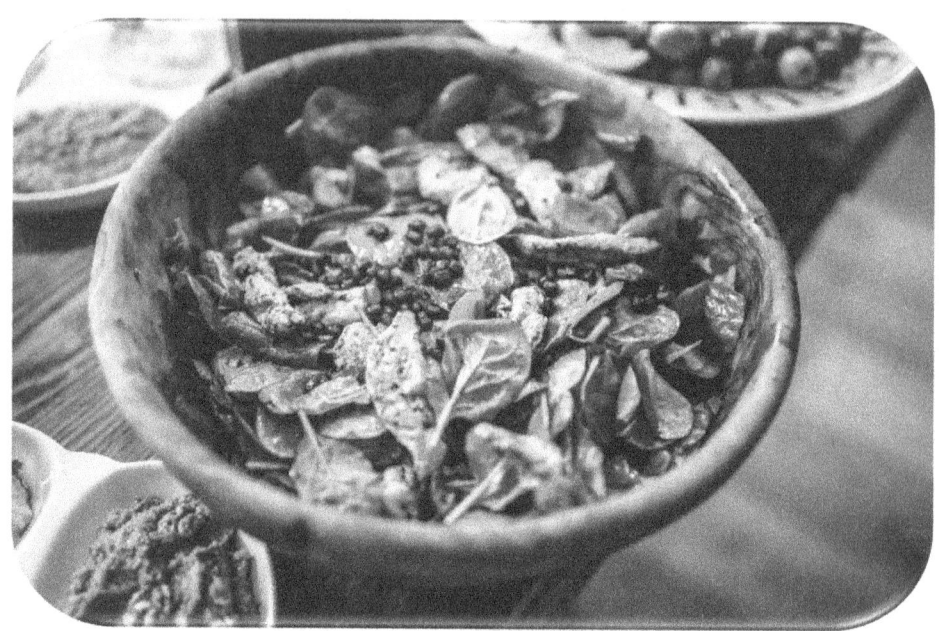

Ingredients:

- 3 cups of chicken meat, cooked, cubed
- 1 cup grapes
- 2 cups fresh spinach
- 1/4 red onion, chopped
- 1 large yellow bell pepper, chopped
- 1/4 cup mayonnaise
- 1 cup pomegranate

Directions:

Put all the salad ingredients into a suitable salad bowl. Toss them well and refrigerate for 1 hour.

Serve.

Nutrition	Calories	Fat	Carbs	Protein	Sodium	Phosphorus	Potassium
	240	8.6g	19.4g	21g	161mg	260mg	269mg

50. Egg Celery Salad

Preparation Time: *10 minutes* | *Cooking Time*: *0 minutes* | *Servings*: *4*

Ingredients:

- 4 eggs, boiled, peeled and chopped
- 1/4 cup celery, chopped
- 1/2 cup sweet onion, chopped
- 2 tablespoons sweet pickle, chopped
- 3 tablespoons mayonnaise
- 1 tablespoon mustard

Directions:

Put all the salad ingredients into a suitable salad bowl. Toss them well and refrigerate for 1 hour.

Serve.

Nutrition	Calories	Fat	Carbs	Protein	Sodium	Phosphorus	Potassium
	134	8.9g	7.4g	6.8g	259mg	357mg	112mg

Conclusion

These recipes are ideal whether you have been diagnosed with a kidney problem or you want to prevent any kidney issue. With regards to your wellbeing and health, it's a smart thought to see your doctor as frequently as conceivable to ensure you don't run into preventable issues that you needn't get. The kidneys are your body's toxin channel (just like the liver), cleaning the blood of remote substances and toxins that are discharged from things like preservatives in food & other toxins.

Thank you for reading and using this book, you have already taken a step towards your success

Best Wishes

CPSIA information can be obtained
at www.ICGtesting.com
Printed in the USA
BVHW040802040321
R11947400001B/R119474PG601388BVX00010B/10